The BHS
Riding and Road Safety Manual

Riding and Roadcraft

12th Edition

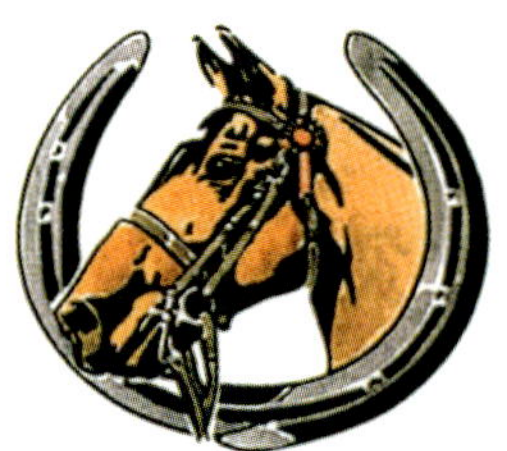

THE BRITISH HORSE SOCIETY

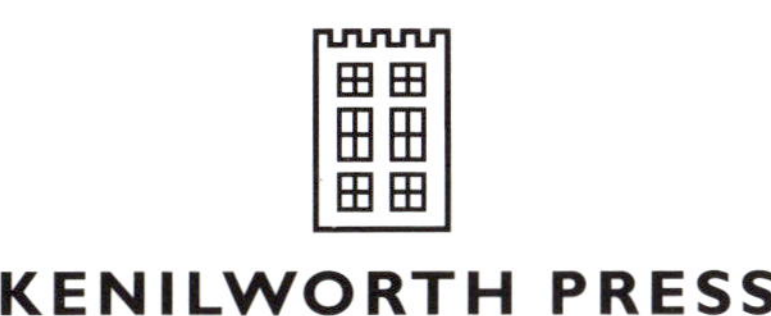

ACKNOWLEDGEMENTS

The British Horse Society wishes to thank:

Dr J M H Lloyd-Parry MA, MB, BChir, for the section on Falls and Injuries; The British Driving Society for work on the driving section; Mrs Ann C Norris originator of the BDS logo; the Side Saddle Association for their advice on the side-saddle section; the *First Aid Manual* published by Dorling Kindersley, from which information is reproduced by kind permission of St John Ambulance, St Andrew's Ambulance Association and British Red Cross; The Official Highway Code Crown copyright 2007; Mr Steven Thompson (Capita Symonds) for his line drawings; Mr Graham Hodgson, Mrs Mary Haimes and Mrs Jo Cameron for their varied contributions; Mrs Sheila Hardy, MAIRSO, BHS Senior Executive Safety, for editorial directions; Mrs Helen Kerry and Mr David Kerry FIRSO, MAIRSO, Dip.ASM, LARSOA for editorial directions and photographic contributions. Above all The Society wish to thank Mrs Carole Mewton for her diligent and painstaking re-writing and formatting of the manual to bring it in to the twenty-first Century.

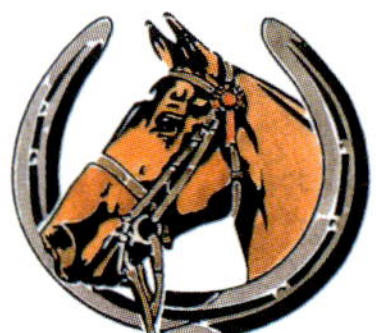

The British Horse Society

Registered Charity No. 210504 and SCO 38516

First published in 1976 as *Ride Safely*
Revised in 1984 as *Ride and Drive Safely*
Revised in 1986 as *Riding and Roadcraft*
7th edition 1989 and revised 1990
8th edition 1993
9th edition 1995; reprinted 1997
10th edition 1999
11th edition 2003
This 12th edition published in the UK in 2009 by Kenilworth Press, an imprint of Quiller Publishing Ltd

British Library Cataloguing-in-Publication Data
A catalogue record for this book is available from the British Library

ISBN 978 1 905693 13 9

A contribution from sales of this publication is made to The British Horse Society's Road Safety Campaign Fund

Printed in Malta by Gutenberg Press Ltd.

Kenilworth Press

An imprint of Quiller Publishing Ltd
Wykey House, Wykey, Shrewsbury, SY4 1JA
Tel: 01939 261616 Fax: 01939 261606
E-mail: info@quillerbooks.com
Website: www.kenilworthpress.co.uk

CONTENTS

FOREWORD

I would recommend this publication to all horse riders and drivers of horse drawn vehicles. It is important that this valuable advice is read along with the Highway Code if you intend to use the highway.

Riders have as much right to use the roads as anyone else and should be able to enjoy riding without fear of dangerous behaviour by other road users. We are making great efforts to educate drivers of the needs of vulnerable road users such as horse riders, under our Road Safety Strategy. I am sure that you will be willing to play your part in helping reduce the number of horse rider related accidents on our roads by following the advice in this manual. I would also encourage you to take The British Horse Society's Riding and Road Safety Test.

Jim Fitzpatrick MP
Parliamentary Under Secretary of State for Transport

INTRODUCTION

Despite everyone's efforts, road traffic accidents involving equines continue to be a hazard faced by all who ride and carriage drive, especially as the speed and volumes of traffic on our roads continues to grow.

It is therefore vitally important that every rider and carriage driver reads this volume thoroughly, heeds the advice given and takes The British Horse Society's Riding and Road Safety Test, as most of us cannot ride without doing some degree of roadwork.

The British Horse Society continues to research means by which we can lessen these incidents and continues to provide the only Riding and Road Safety Test that is recognised by the Department for Transport.

Every person who rides a horse on the road, should train for, and take, The British Horse Society Riding and Road Safety Test which will teach them the correct way to ride safely on today's busy roads.

Patrick Print FBHS
Chairman
The British Horse Society

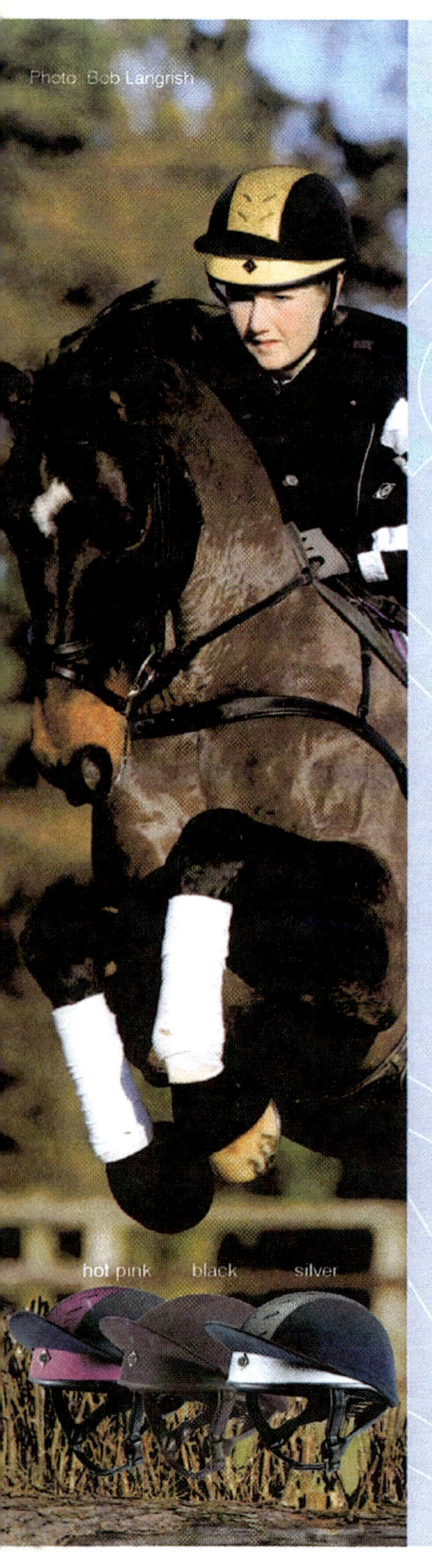
Photo: Bob Langrish
hot pink
black
silver

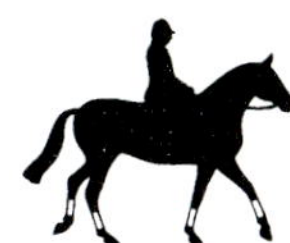

1. ARE YOU READY FOR THE ROAD?

How to prepare

Make sure you have a copy of the current Highway Code and take time to study it.

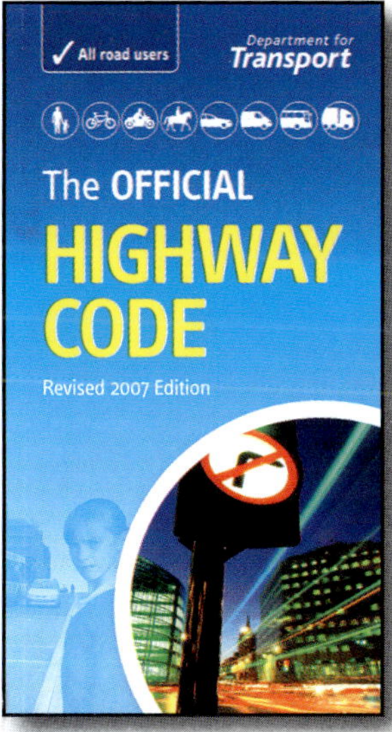

> **Highway Code Rule 52**
> Before you take your horse on the road you should
> - make sure you can control your horse.

All road users have a duty of care to each other and must have a thorough understanding of the current edition of The Official Highway Code.

(NB: The highlighted Highway Code sections in this Manual do not quote the Highway Code in full)

- You should be a competent rider before riding on the public highway.
- It is recommended that special training in road skills is taken.
- This edition of the Riding and Roadcraft Manual must be read in conjunction with the Highway Code.
- The hooves and shoes of your horse should be kept in good condition. They should be regularly checked by a Registered Farrier.
- Fluorescent/reflective equipment for both horse and rider are necessary.

Be safe-Be seen
Always use fluorescent/reflective leg-bands, tabards and hat bands/covers

Insurance

Riders and horse owners are strongly advised to hold public liability insurance. This insurance is automatically extended to Gold Members of The British Horse Society.

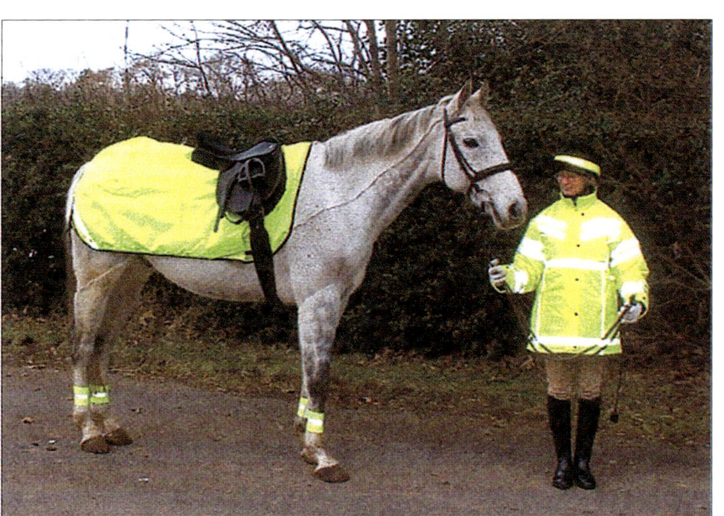

Under certain circumstances a rider may be considered liable if their horse/pony causes harm to a person or person's property and may be required to pay considerable damages.

Riders should be wary of using tabards with words such as **Caution Young Horse/ Novice Rider.**

Fluorescent material can be seen three seconds sooner by other road users.

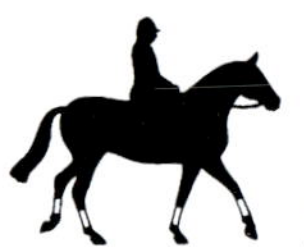

2. TACK, EQUIPMENT, HATS, FOOTWEAR AND CLOTHING

Tack and equipment

Highway Code Rule 52
Before you take a horse on to the road, you should
- ensure all tack fits well and is in good condition.
- ...Never ride a horse without both a saddle and bridle.

- Flexible/supple tack adds to the comfort of your horse.
- Regularly check the leather, stitching and buckles for wear.
- Check that the stirrup bar is in the down position.
- Always use fluorescent/reflective leg-bands. These should be fitted on all four legs above the fetlock joints.

  (NOTE: These leg-bands are compulsory for the BHS Riding and Road Safety Test.)

Stirrup irons

- These should be the correct size for your foot. As a guide a minimum of 6mm (1/4 inch) clearance is recommended. This is on both sides at the ball of the foot when in the stirrup iron.

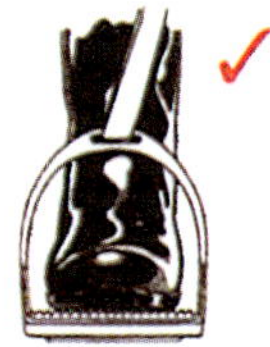

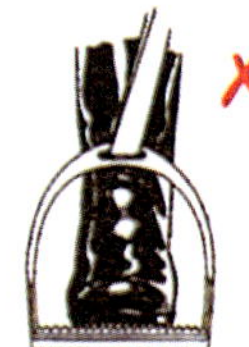

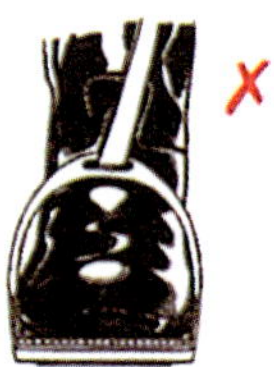

Hats

Highway Code Rule 49
- Children under the age of 14 MUST wear a helmet which complies with the Regulation. It MUST be fastened securely.
- Other riders should also follow these requirements.

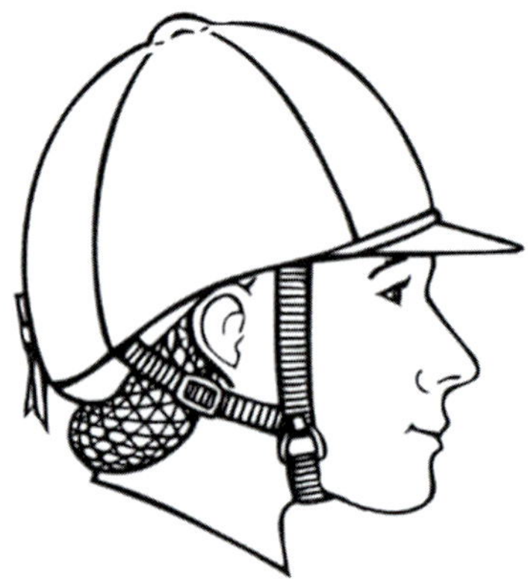

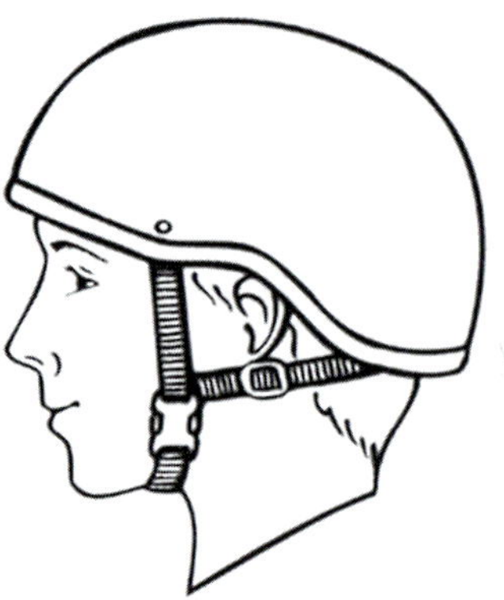

Hats must be correctly fitted, secured with a minimum three point harness and comply with the Regulations. For maximum protection headgear should conform to at least one of the following:-

PAS 015 (94),
ASTM F1163
SNELL E2001
BSEN 1384:1997
(EN1384:1996*)
*preferably with Quality Assurance Mark such as BSi Kitemark or SEI mark

(NOTE: These standards are mandatory for the BHS Riding and Road Safety Test. The hat worn should be the rider's own hat, correctly fitted and secured with a minimum three point harness.)

These are the current recommendations of The British Horse Society. This information is correct at the time of printing.

Footwear

Highway Code Rule 50
- You should wear boots or shoes with hard soles and heels.

- Boots/shoes with through soles and small heels should be worn. (Repaired half soled boots/shoes can catch in the stirrup irons). Soft soled footwear, trainers and some Wellington boots are dangerous for riding and should not be worn.
- Some 'Yard' boots are also unacceptable for riding as they do not have appropriate tread. (Your Riding and Road Safety Trainer should be able to advise you on what is safe.)

(NOTE: Soft footwear e.g. trainers are not acceptable for The BHS Riding and Road Safety Test.)

Highway Code Rule 50
You should wear
- Light-coloured or fluorescent clothing in daylight.
- Reflective clothing if you have to ride at night or in poor visibility.

Riders' clothing

- Wearing light-coloured and/or reflective/ fluorescent gloves will help make your hand signals clearer.
- Long-sleeved clothing may help to protect a rider's arm if a rider falls or is thrown from their horse. Short-sleeved clothing should be avoided and is not acceptable for the Riding and Road Safety Test.
- Fluorescent tabards, hat bands/covers should be worn.

(NOTE: Dark coloured gloves are not permitted for The BHS Riding and Road Safety Test.)

!
PROTECTIVE HELMET
Riding gloves
Long-soled boots
Whip
Tack in good condition
Horse correctly shod, hooves correctly trimmed
Reflective/ fluorescent clothing

2A. THE HIGHWAY CODE

Make sure you have a copy of the current Highway Code – and take time time to study it.

Statutory rules affecting riders

By law:

You **MUST NOT** deliberately ride, lead or drive your horse:

- on a footpath by the side of any road made or set apart for the use of pedestrians (England and Wales).
- on a footway, footpath or cycle track unless there is a right to do so (Scotland).

Children under fourteen **MUST** wear a properly secured approved safety helmet.

REMEMBER:

LARGE VEHICLES NEED A GREATER DISTANCE TO STOP. BEWARE OF AIR BRAKES.

BE AWARE:

AIR-BRAKES ON HEAVY VEHICLES MAY BLOW OFF AT ANY TIME – THIS IS BEYOND THE DRIVER'S CONTROL.

REMEMBER:

ALL VEHICLES NEED MORE DISTANCE TO STOP WHEN THE ROAD SURFACE IS WET OR ICY OR COVERED IN SNOW (See 'Dangerous Road Conditions', page 33 for further advice).

Traffic light signals

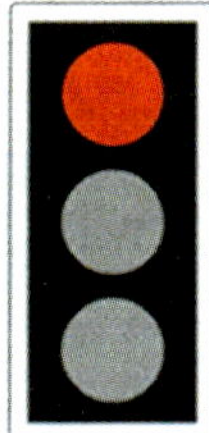

RED means 'Stop'. Wait behind the stop line on the carriageway.

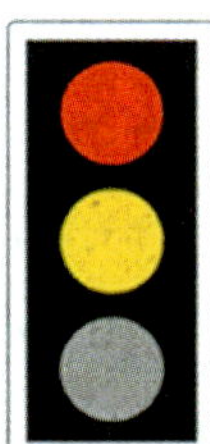

RED AND AMBER also means 'Stop'. Prepare to move off but do not pass through or start until GREEN shows.

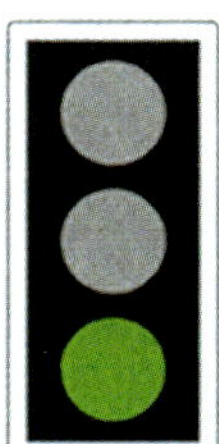

GREEN means you may go on if the way is clear. Take special care if you intend to turn left or right and give way to pedestrians who are crossing.

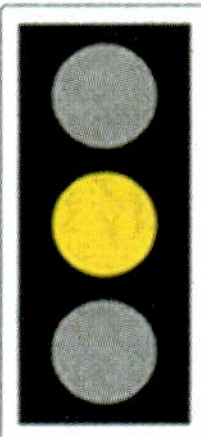

AMBER means 'Stop' at the stop line. You may go on only if the AMBER appears after you have crossed the stop line.

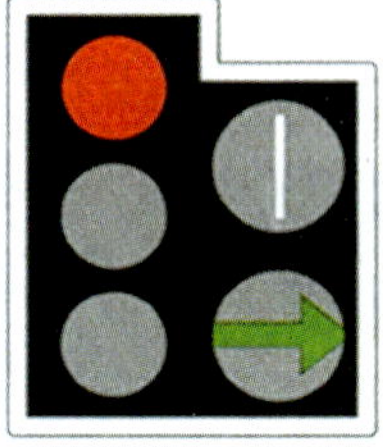

A GREEN ARROW → may be provided in addition to the full green signal if movement in a certain direction is allowed before or after the full green phase. If the way is clear you may go but only in the direction shown by the arrow. You may do this whatever other lights may be showing.

Flashing red lights

At level crossings, lifting bridges, airfields, fire stations.

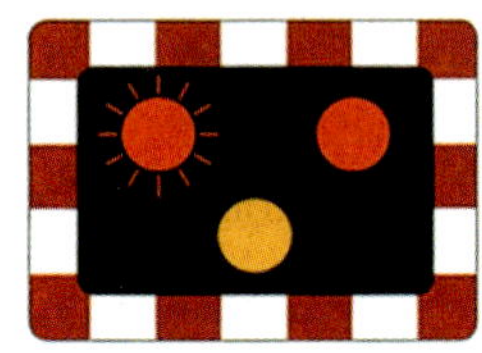

Alternately flashing red lights mean YOU MUST STOP.

Road markings across the carriageway

Give way to traffic on major road

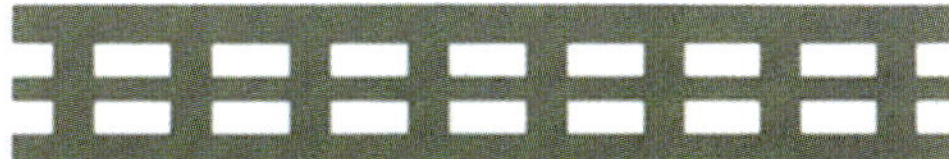

Give way to traffic on major road

Give way to traffic from right in roundabout

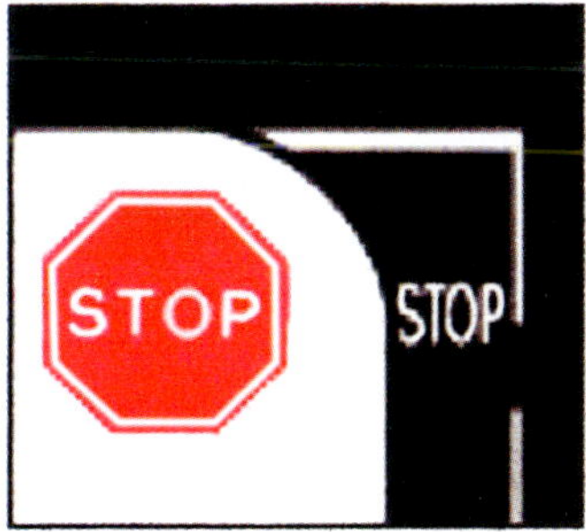

Stop line at 'Stop' sign

Give way to traffic from right at mini-roundabout

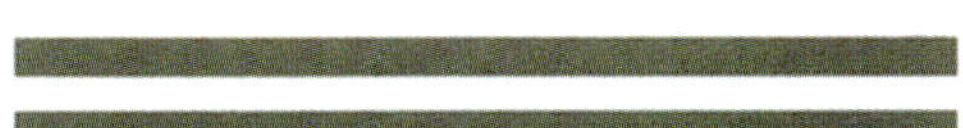

Stop line at signals or police control

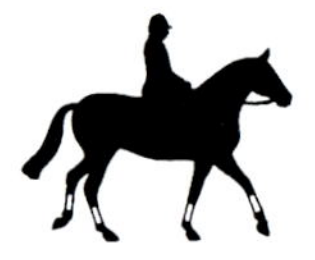

3 CONSIDERATION, COURTESY AND ROAD AWARENESS

Riders should:

- Understand that good manners are a necessary part of their road skills.
- Thank those who show consideration. This may be done verbally, with a nod, a smile or where safe, a hand raised in thanks.
- Ensure acknowledgements are clear, generous, timely and visible to the driver.
- Pass riders and pedestrians at a walk.
- Ask permission from riders and pedestrians in front of them before passing.
- Take particular care when passing pedestrians. They may be frightened of horses. A friendly acknowledgement will help to reassure them.

Road awareness

Highway Code Rules 53, 105, 109, 111 and 148

Before riding off or turning, look behind you to make sure it is safe, then give a clear arm signal.

- You MUST obey signals given by police officers, traffic officers.......
- You MUST obey all traffic light signals and traffic signs giving orders.......
- Never assume that flashing headlights is a signal inviting you to proceed.......
- Safe driving and riding needs concentration.

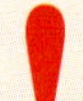

Be aware, look, listen and <u>think</u> ahead

Approach bends and corners at a walk. The road surface may be slippery. Be particularly aware of traffic both in front and behind. On left-hand bends and turns, always check over your left shoulder for any pedestrians or cyclists approaching on your near side.

Be alert for possible hazards particularly from behind. Look around regularly to check the changing road situation.

Be aware of bad weather and changing road conditions.

Listen for approaching cars and cyclists and other noises that may cause your horse to be startled.

Look and listen for children playing near the road. They may well run out unexpectedly from between parked cars. Uncontrolled and barking dogs may frighten your horse.

!

REMEMBER
Expect the unexpected.
Establish eye contact with other road users.
Never move unless it is safe.
Never take a chance – remember your 'life-saver' look.
Note: an informed driver is usually a more understanding driver.
BE ROAD AWARE – STAY SAFE

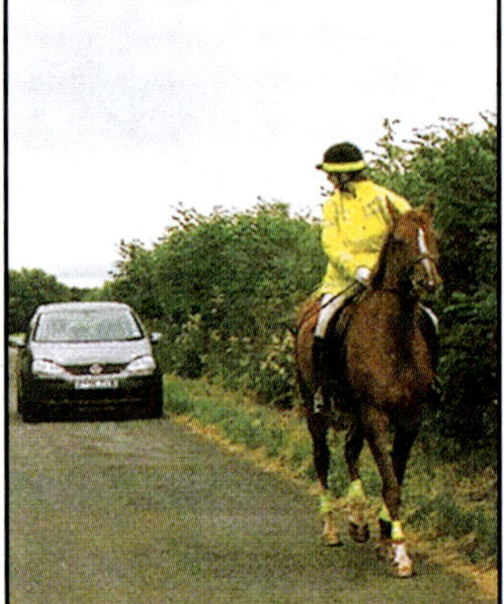

Rider demonstrating good observations

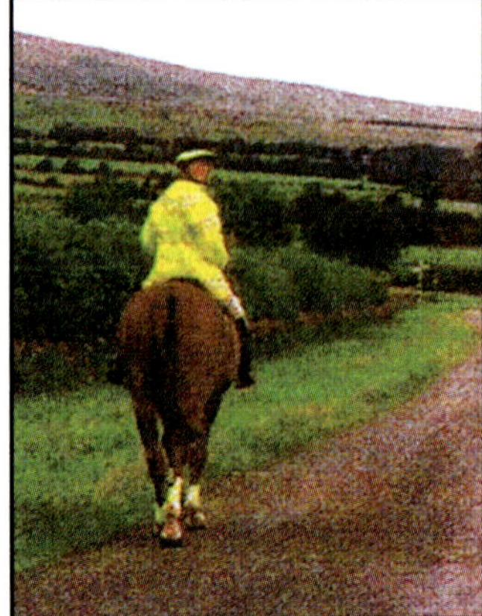

'I've seen you'

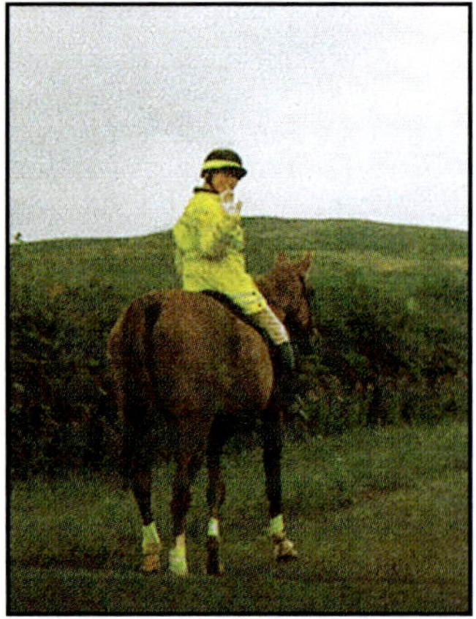

'Thank you for waiting'

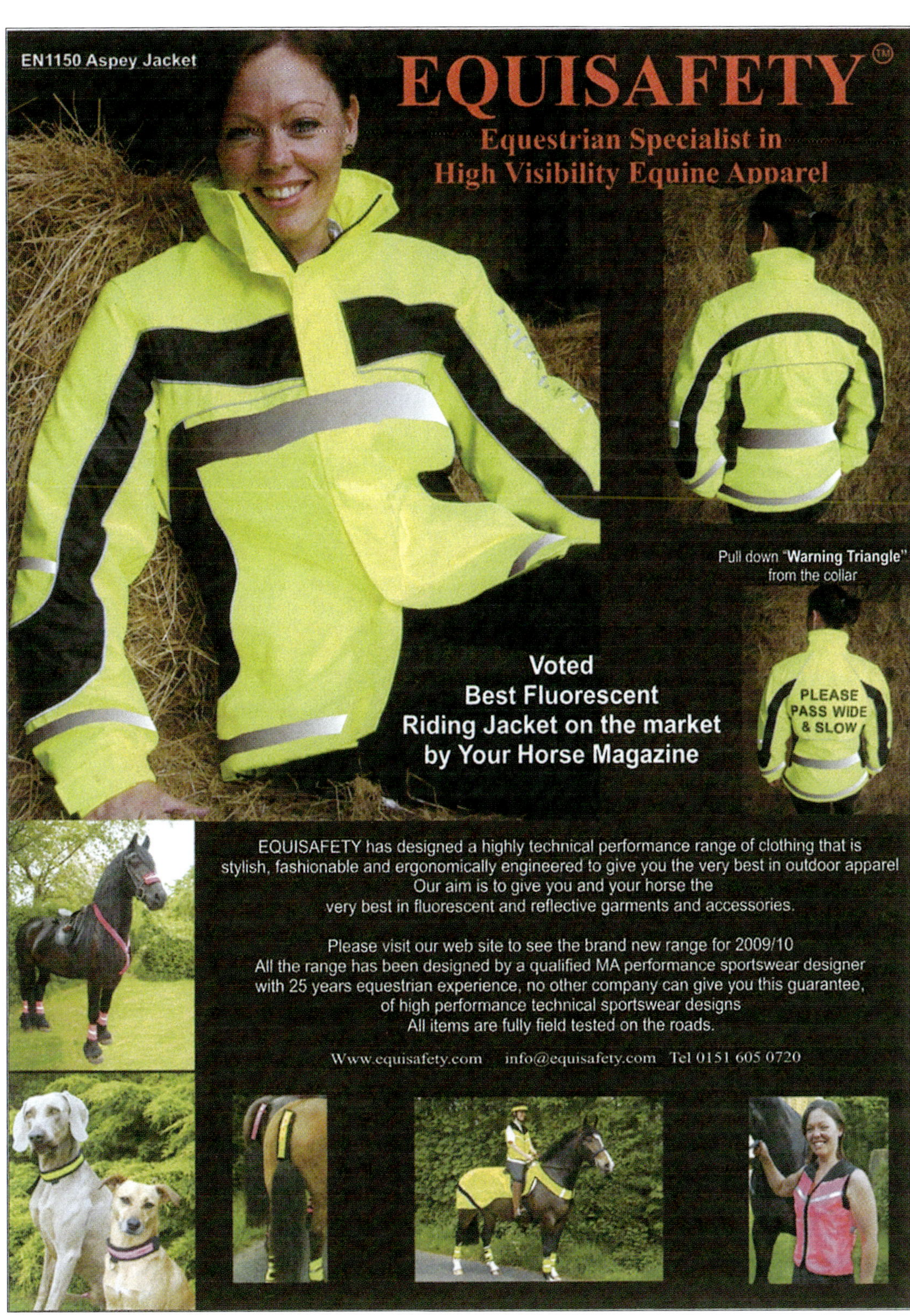
EN1150 Aspey Jacket
EQUISAFETY
Equestrian Specialist in
High Visibility Equine Apparel
Pull down "Warning Triangle" from the collar
PLEASE PASS WIDE & SLOW
Voted
Best Fluorescent
Riding Jacket on the market
by Your Horse Magazine
EQUISAFETY has designed a highly technical performance range of clothing that is stylish, fashionable and ergonomically engineered to give you the very best in outdoor apparel
Our aim is to give you and your horse the very best in fluorescent and reflective garments and accessories.
Please visit our web site to see the brand new range for 2009/10
All the range has been designed by a qualified MA performance sportswear designer with 25 years equestrian experience, no other company can give you this guarantee, of high performance technical sportswear designs
All items are fully field tested on the roads.
Www.equisafety.com info@equisafety.com Tel 0151 605 0720

4. ROAD SKILLS

Highway Code Rules 53, 54 and 103
- keep both hands on the reins unless you are signalling.
- keep both feet in the stirrups.
- never ride more than two abreast and ride in single file on narrow roads and when riding round bends.
- not carry anything which might affect your balance or get tangled up with the reins.
- You MUST NOT take a horse onto a foot path or pavement…
- give clear signals in plenty of time…

Observation

- Carry out observations. Look all round, listen and assess your surroundings.
- When safe give appropriate signal to inform other road users of your intentions.
- Carry out **'life-saver'** observations – looking, listening and assessing your surroundings.
- When safe carry out your manoeuvre – be cautious but not hesitant. Taking too long to complete an action can turn you into a hazard.
- To look behind turn from the waist, keep both hands on the reins.
- A **'life-saver look'** is the look you usually give over your right shoulder, after you have made all your checks and immediately before you move off just to confirm that is is safe.
- **Look, listen, look again before making any signal**

Road positioning

Highway Code Rule 53
- Keep to the left.

- Ride on the left of the road but not hugging the kerb.
- Ride straight and use your leg aids to help prevent the horse from moving sideways or swinging his hindquarters into the road.
- Reins must be at the correct length to control the horse.
- Take a good position at junctions so you can see traffic approaching from any direction.
- Avoid potholes, manhole covers and drains which could be slippery.

Defensive riding

On occasions, such as a narrow lane with no verge, it may be necessary, sensible and safe to take up the amount of road normally used by a motor vehicle. A rider should not obstruct other road users.

ALWAYS
- Thank considerate drivers.
- Be ready to move out of the way quickly.
- Be aware of blind bends – and the changes in road conditions.

Road junctions

Highway Code Rules 170 and 53
Take extra care at junctions.
You should…
- keep to the left.
- watch out for pedestrians crossing…
- not assume, when waiting at a junction, that a vehicle coming from the right and signalling left will actually turn. Wait and make sure.

- Have you allowed enough time and space to cross the road **safely?**
- Keep your horse under control.
- Do not move off until it is **safe**.

OBSERVE – the traffic situation **thoroughly.**
ALWAYS – look right and left when crossing the road.
SIGNAL – **clearly** and **positively.**
REMEMBER – your **Life-saver look.**
BOTH HANDS – should be on the reins unless signalling.

IN SHORT:

- LOOK
- SIGNAL
- LOOK – AND IF SAFE –
- DO IT

Highway Code Rules 53, 103 and 215

- Before riding off or turning, look behind you to make sure it is safe, then give a clear arm signal.
- Signals warn and inform other road users of your intended actions.
- ...Look out for horse riders' and horse drivers' signals and heed a request to slow down or stop. Take great care and treat all horses as a potential hazard; they can be unpredictable, despite the efforts of their rider/driver.

- Remember a signal is not a guarantee of your safety.
- It should be clear and not confuse.
- Both hands should be on the reins before moving off.
- The whip should not be used to make a signal.

How to signal:

- Riders must look before signalling.
- To signal right or left, the arm must be fully extended at shoulder height.
- The fingers and thumb should be closed together and the palm of the hand should be facing forwards.
- The signal should be held long enough to inform others of your intent and repeated as necessary dependent on road conditions and behaviour of your horse.

To signal with your right hand:

- Keep the whip on the right hand side of the horse.
- Tuck the whip under the left hand thumb.
- The right hand is then free to make the signal.

Note

If you are certain that there is no one to see and take benefit from your signal, then it is not necessary to make one. The safest place for your hands is on the reins.

Never signal with a whip

Signals

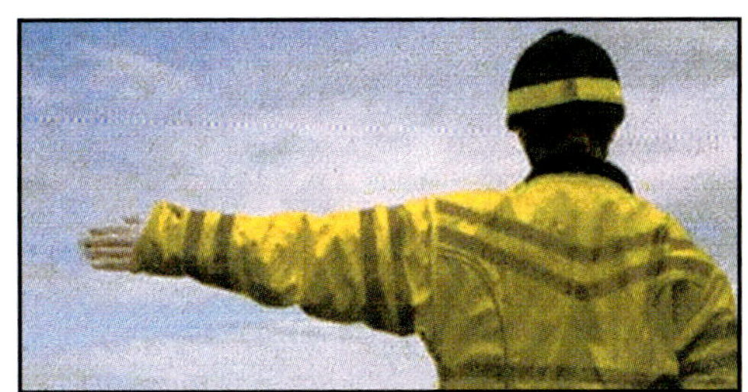

Turning left

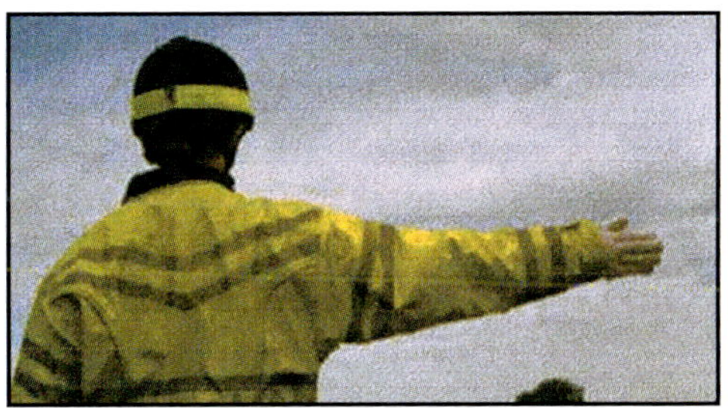

Turning right

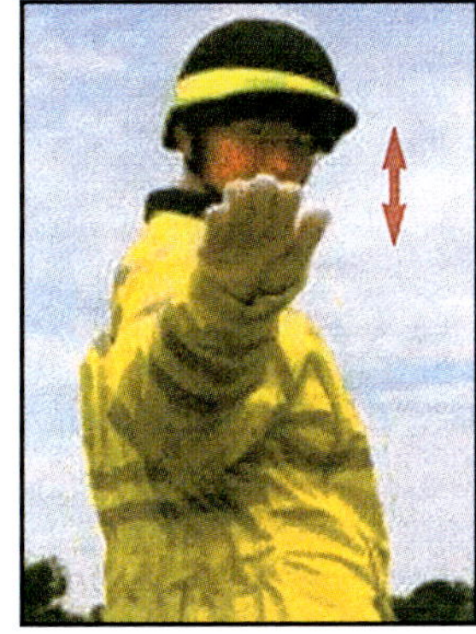

Advisory signals

To request a road user to slow down, turn in the saddle to face them. The right arm is extended with the palm facing down and moved slowly up and down. This may be repeated if necessary.

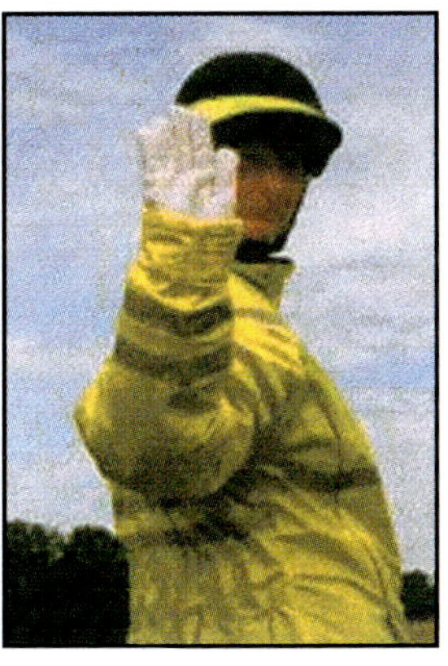

To request a road user to stop, turn in the saddle to face them. The right arm is extended with the palm facing the driver. A second signal may be necessary in certain situations.

5. EMERGENCY DISMOUNT, LEAD AND REMOUNT

Highway Code Rule 53

- Keep to the left.
- Keep a horse you are leading to your left.

Dismount only if it is really necessary. It is usually safer to stay on the horse's back.

Dismount either on the near side or the off side, which ever is the easiest, safest and quickest for you.

Emergency dismount

- Look behind, and find a safe place if possible off the highway. The horse should be positioned with its quarters slightly in.
- Look again before taking both feet out of the stirrups. Cross one stirrup over in front of the saddle (on the horse's shoulder). If dismounting on the left transfer the whip into the left hand before dismounting.
- **Dismount.**
- Place the other stirrup over the seat of the saddle. The stirrups leathers are then not crossed over each other.
- Check all around for traffic.
- Quickly but carefully, the rider needs to put themselves **between the horse and the traffic**.
- Take the reins over the horse's head **unless the horse is wearing a running martingale**.

Lead

- Look behind, signal if necessary and if clear with the reins in both hands and whip in the right hand, walk on. Position yourself at the horse's head. **Place yourself between your horse and the traffic**.
- Keep looking all around whilst leading.
- Find a safe place to remount.

Remount

- Check it is safe.
- Take down the off side stirrup **carefully** (if mounting from the near side).
- Put the reins back over the horse's head.
- Check it is safe before moving to the near side.
- Check the girth.
- Take down the near side stirrup.
- Place the whip in left hand.
- Remount transfer the whip back into the right hand and look all around before moving off.

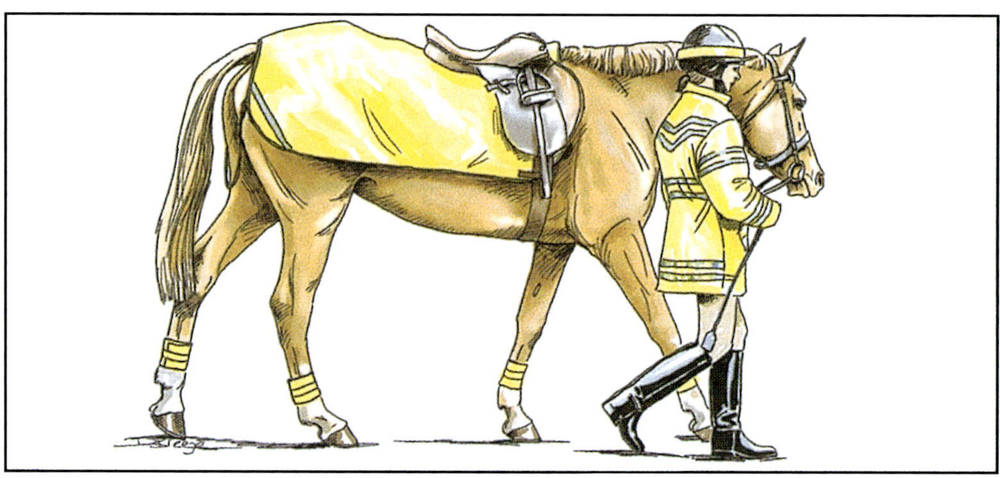

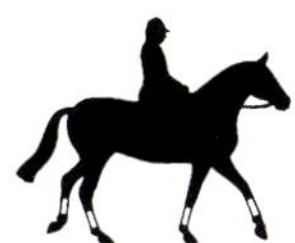

6. STATIONARY VEHICLES, OBSTRUCTIONS, DANGEROUS/FRIGHTENING HAZARDS

Highway Code Rule 163

You should...

- overtake only when it is safe and legal to do so.
- not get too close to the vehicle you intend to overtake.

You should:

- Keep to the left and look behind in good time.
- You may need to stop and wait for traffic.
- When safe, signal right, give a 'life-saver' look and move out gradually to pass the obstacle.
- Be aware of pedestrians walking out from in front of the obstacle.
- If passing a vehicle allow enough room for a car door to be opened. Check, and listen for. sudden movement or noise from within the car.
- Move back gradually to the near side of the road allowing safe clearance of the obstacle.

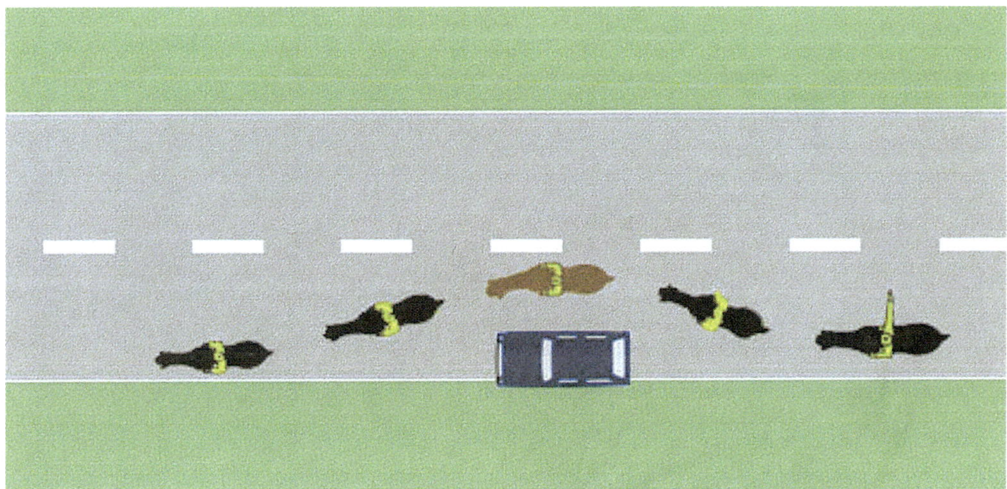

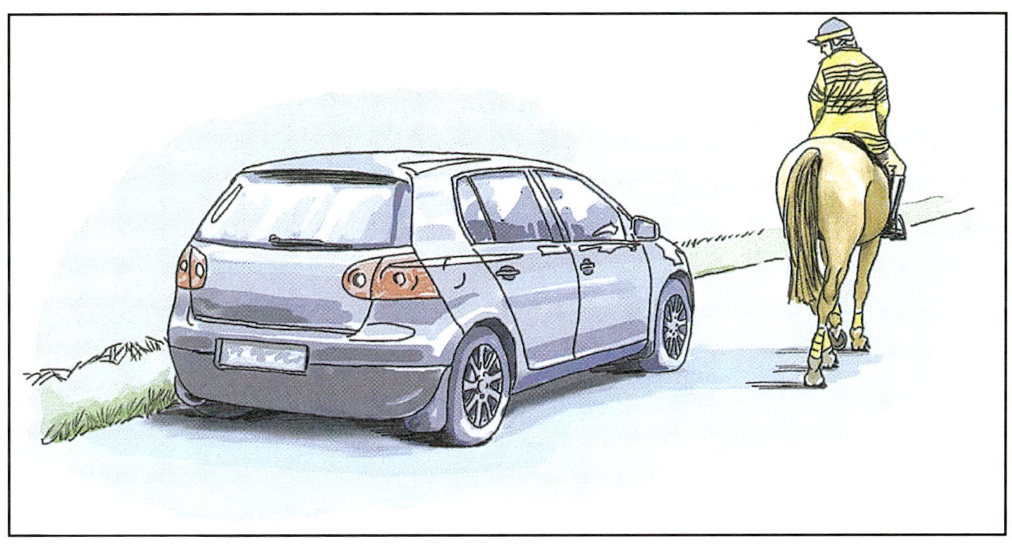

Road works

These should be ridden as if passing an obstacle. If your horse shows resistance then you may need to find a different route instead of trying to force your horse to pass.

Dangerous/noisy/frightening hazards

These include road drills, compressors, hedge cutters etc.

- Stop a safe distance away if traffic is approaching.
- Try to catch the operator's attention and thank them if they are helpful.
- If your horse will not go forward and you are in company, ask for a lead from another horse.
- If you are by yourself, consider using an alternative route.

Think ahead, if you know of a problem, take a different route. The road is not the place to school your horse.

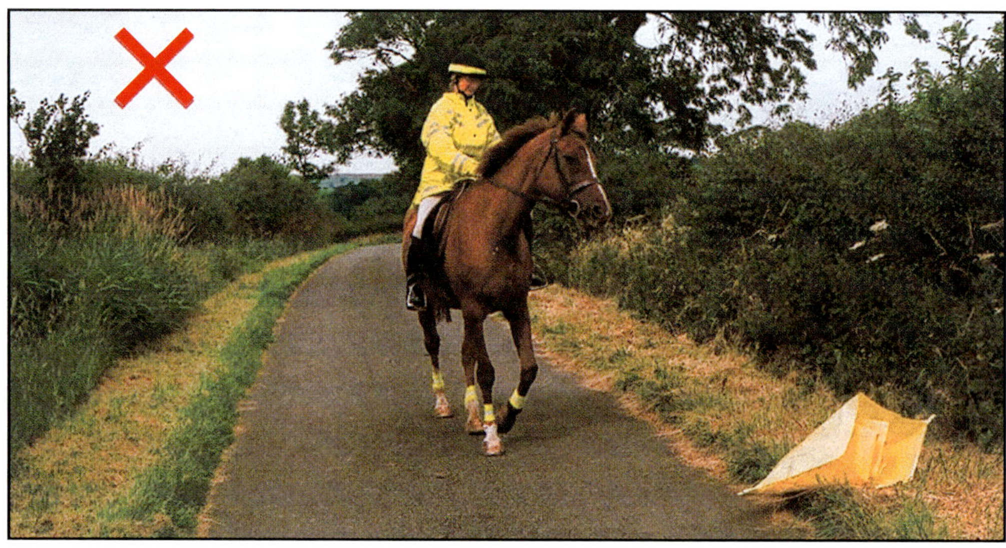

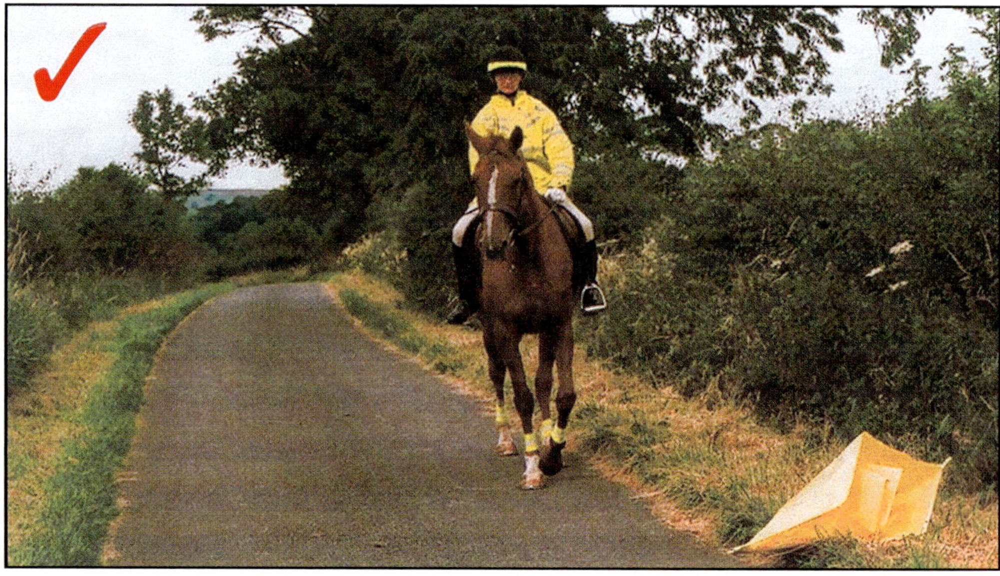

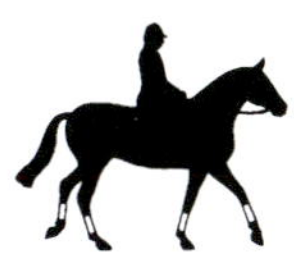

7. LEADING A HORSE ON FOOT AND LEADING A HORSE WHEN MOUNTED

When leading a horse on the public highway whether mounted or dismounted, the led horse should always wear a bridle.

Highway Code Rules 51 and 53

- ...If you are leading a horse at night, carry a light in your right hand, showing white to the front and red to the rear...
- keep a horse you are leading to your left.

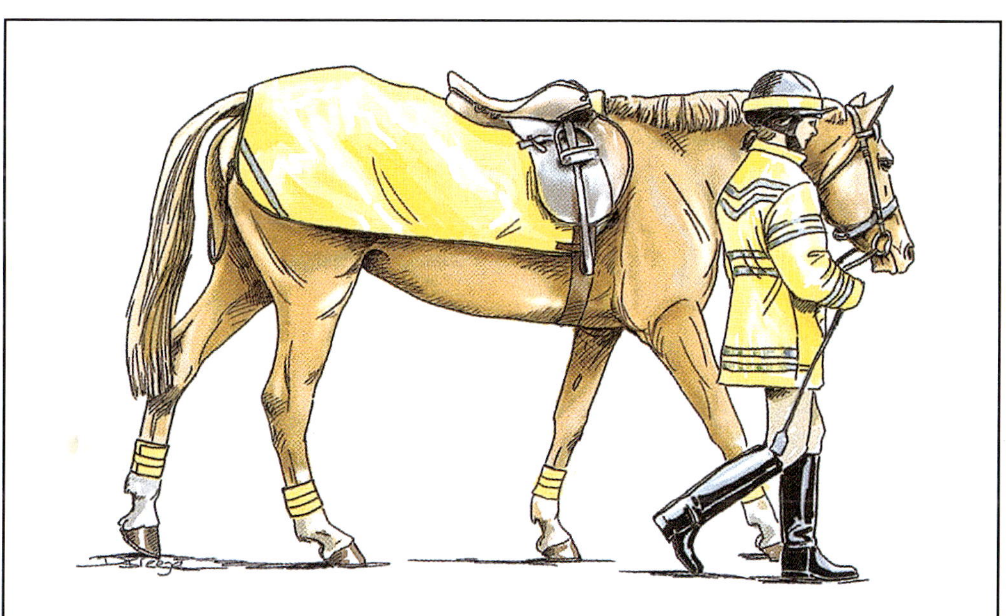

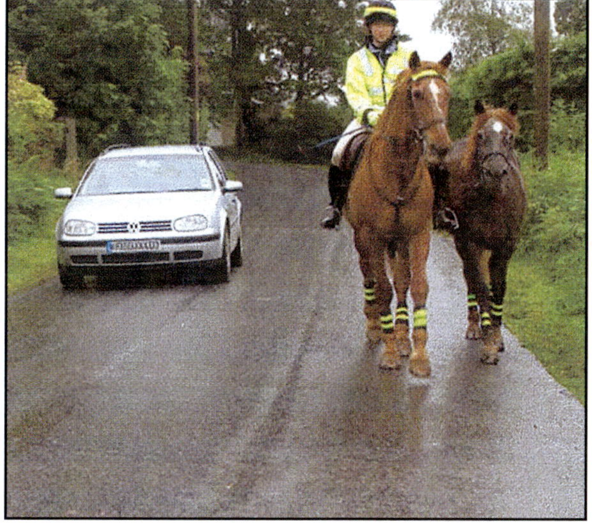

Leading a horse on foot

On the public highway keep to the left, **place yourself between your horse and the traffic** and make sure that both you and your horse are wearing reflective and fluorescent clothing. Your horse should wear reflective leg bands fitted on all four legs above the fetlocks.

Leading a horse when mounted

- Keep to the left of the road.
- Keep the horse you are leading to your left, on the inside.
- **The led horse should wear a bridle** with the reins passed through the bit rings. (See also Section II.)

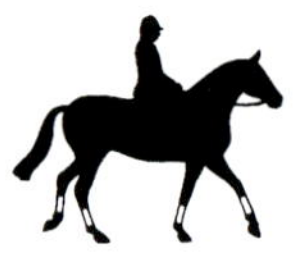

8. RIGHT TURNS, LEFT TURNS, CROSS ROADS, TRAFFIC LIGHTS AND ROUNDABOUTS

T-Junctions Minor to Major

Left Turn

Highway Code Rules 182 and 183

- …watch out for traffic coming up on your left.
  When turning
- keep as close to the left as is safe and practicable.

1. Look all around.
2. Signal in good time if safe.
3. Check over right shoulder.
4. If clear and safe, ride on.
   Watch for traffic as you make your turn. If you have to stop for traffic at the junction:
   - Carefully check for traffic.
   - You may have to signal again.
   - Look all around.
   - Check over left shoulder.
   - Check over right shoulder.
   - Move off when safe, keep looking and listening.
   - Keep to the left.

When on your new route keep checking for traffic.

Remember your **'life-saver'** look.

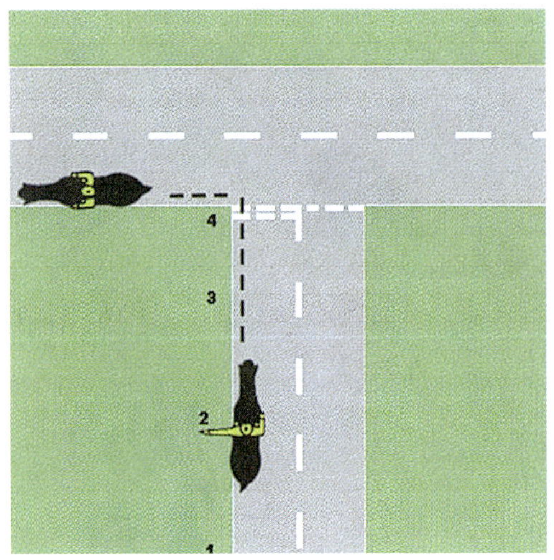

Right Turn

Highway Code Rule 180

- Do not cut the corner. Take great care when turning into a main road; you will need to watch for traffic in both directions and wait for a safe gap

1. Look all around.
2. Signal if safe.
3. Check over right shoulder.
4. If clear and safe, ride on.
   Watch for traffic as you make your turn. If you have to stop for traffic at the junction:
   - Carefully check for traffic.
   - You may need to signal again.
   - Look all around.
   - Check over right shoulder.
   - Move off when safe, keep looking and listening.
   - Walk straight across the road. Do not ride diagonally across.

When on your new route keep checking for traffic.

Remember your **'life-saver'** look.

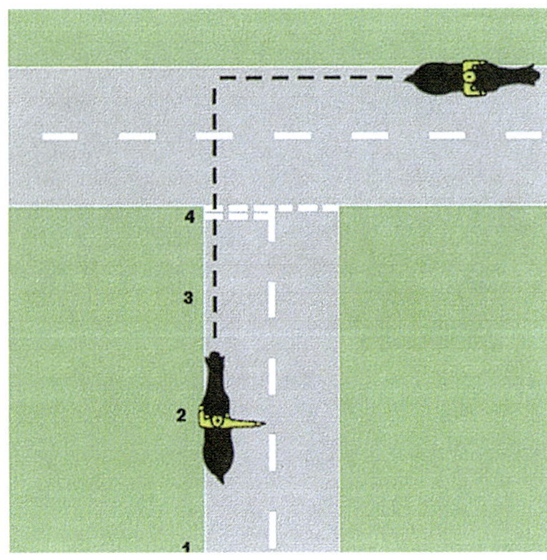

Flared Junctions Minor to Major

Left Turn

You should ride this in the same order as the left turn at a T- junction. **A safe position at this junction is very important.**

- Place yourself at right angles to the **Give Way/Stop** line.
- Do not keep too close to the kerb.
- Make sure that traffic can not pass you on your left.
- Make sure that traffic behind can see you (See diagram).

Remember your **'life-saver'** look.

Be safe Be seen

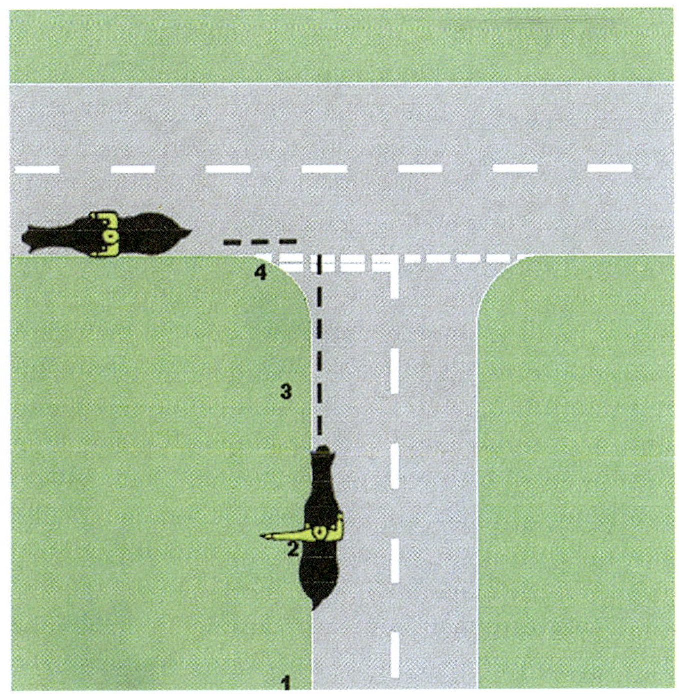

Right Turn

You should ride this in the same order as the right turn at a T- junction. **A safe position at this junction is very important.**

- Place yourself at right angles to the **Give Way/Stop** line.
- Try to make sure that traffic cannot pass you on your left.
- Make sure that traffic behind can see you (See diagram).

Remember your **'life-saver'** look.

Be safe Be seen

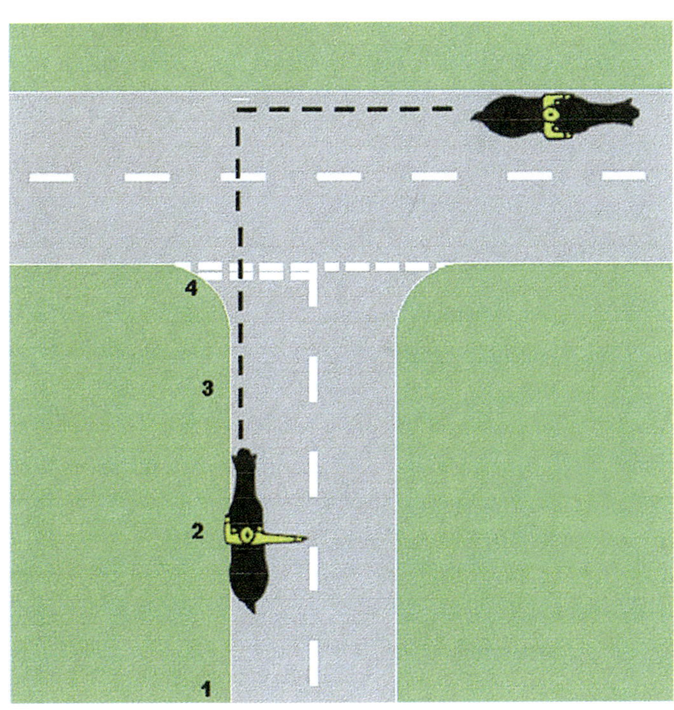

Major Road to Minor Road

Left Turn

1. Look all around.
2. Signal in good time if safe.
3. Check over right shoulder.
4. Keep moving, keep looking.
   - Check over left shoulder.
   - Check over right shoulder.
   - Keep as close to the left as is safe when turning.

Remember your **'life-saver'** look.

Be safe Be seen

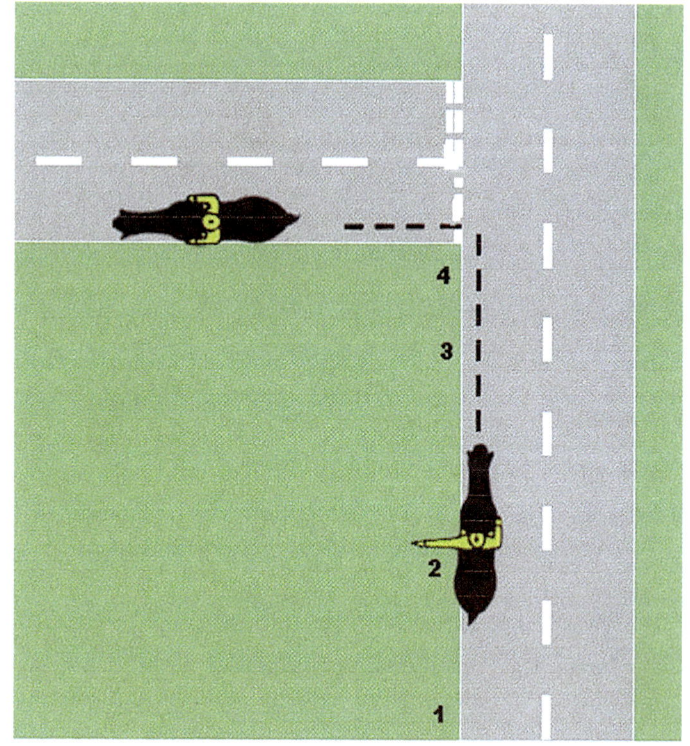

Right Turn

1. Look all around.
2. Signal if it is safe.
3. Check over right shoulder.
4. Look, listen, carefully check for traffic.
5. Opposite the junction, check behind. Make sure your actions are under-stood. If safe turn, straight across the road. Keep looking.

Note
If the traffic does not allow you to safely make the turn.

- Either, wait opposite the junction until it is clear.
- Or, ride on along the road. Make a U-turn when it is safe (as described on the following pages).

Remember your **'life-saver'** look

Be safe Be seen

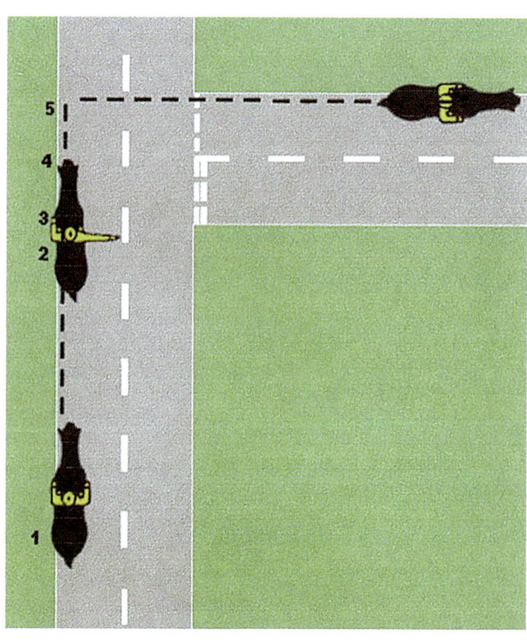

Crossroads and U-turns

Turn Left

You should ride this in the same order as the T- junction/ flared junction.

- Make sure your actions are understood.
- Be aware of traffic coming from the opposite junction which could be turning right.

Remember your **'life-saver'** look.

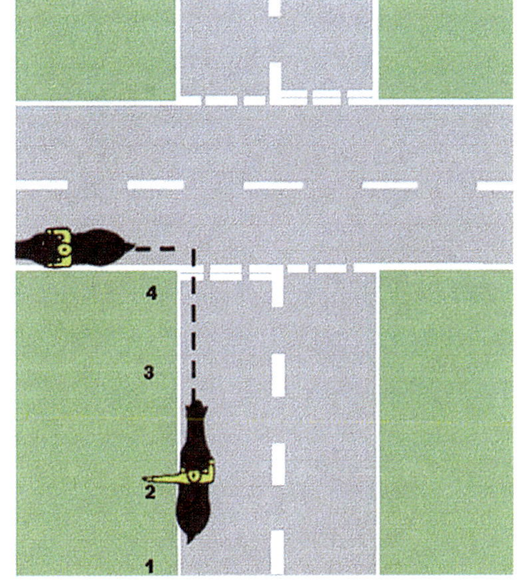

Turn Right/Straight Ahead

You should ride this in the same order as the T- junction/flared junction.

- Make sure your actions are understood.
- If turning right, be aware of traffic coming from the opposite junction which may turn in front of you or over-take you to drive straight ahead. Take a last look before you actually turn across the road.
- If riding straight ahead, keep looking all around as traffic may cut across you. Check the traffic carefully.

Note
If you cannot make your right turn safely, take the alternative route as shown.

Remember your **'life-saver'** look.

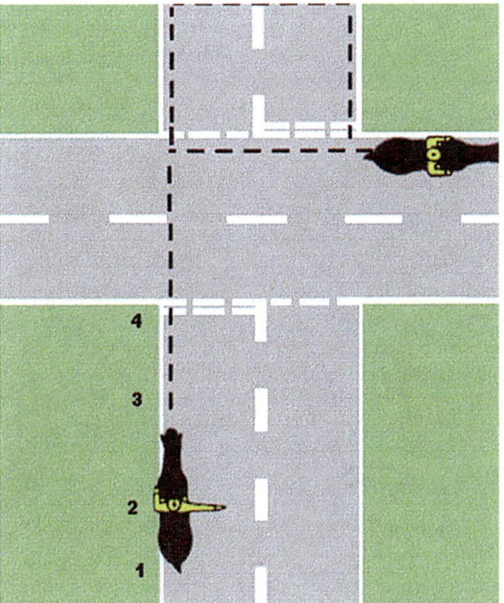

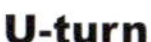

U-turn

If road conditions make it unsafe to turn across the flow of traffic it may be necessary to ride in a different direction until safe to make a U-turn. To execute a U-turn carry out effective observations, signal your intent and when safe, turn across the road and ride back to your chosen route.

Stay calm, take extra care, be sensible be safe

Traffic lights – These may have filter lanes

Highway Code Rule 109

- You MUST obey all traffic light signals…

Thoroughly observe the traffic situation. Beware of vehicles crossing through lights on amber.
At green, Go – if it is safe to do so.

Turn Left

1. Look all around.
2. Signal. Be prepared to stop.
3. Check behind.
4. If the signal shows green and it is safe, ride on, keep looking.
   If the signal is showing amber on its own or red, stop behind the line. Check the traffic.
   - When red and amber show, look behind. Signal again.
   - When green appears, look all around.
   - Check over right shoulder.
   - Move off if it is safe, checking to your left.
   - Do not hesitate, keep moving.

Remember your **'life-saver'** look.

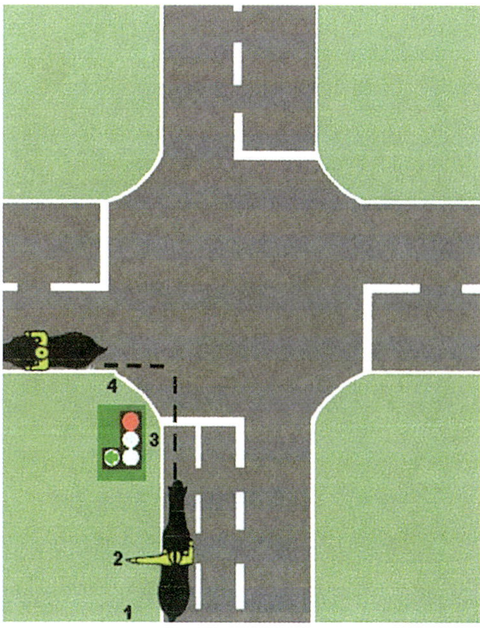

Turn Right/Straight Ahead

1. Look all around.
2. Signal if turning right. Be prepared to stop.
3. Check behind.
4. If the signal shows green and it is safe, ride on, keep looking.
   If the signal is showing amber on its own or red, stop behind the line. Check the traffic.
   - When red and amber show look behind. Signal again if turning right.
   - When green appears, look all around.
   - Check over right shoulder.
   - Move off if it is safe. Keep looking.
   - If turning right, make your turn as shown in diagram. If riding straight across continue as shown in the diagram.
   - Do not hesitate, keep moving.

Remember your **'life-saver'** look.

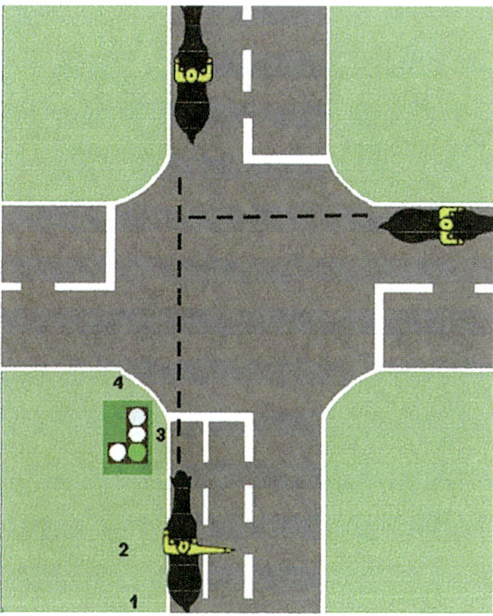

Some lane markings for a right turn may take you to the centre of the road. This may be unsafe as traffic will be on both sides. It would be safer to ride straight on, make a turn across the road and ride back to make a left turn to return to your intended road route.

Roundabouts

Highway Code Rule 55

Avoid roundabouts wherever possible. If you use them you should

- keep to the left and watch out for vehicles crossing your path to leave or join the roundabout.

1. On approaching a roundabout keep to the left and look behind.
2. Give a **'life-saver'** look before stopping (see note*).
   - Look right.
   - Check to the left.
   - Give a **'life-saver'** look behind.
   - Move off, if safe, onto the roundabout.
3. Look over your right shoulder.
4. Signal right as you approach each junction where you are not leaving the roundabout (i.e. turning left).
   - Look behind and look left as you cross the exit.
5. Just before reaching your exit, look all around, signal left, check behind, and make your turn.

*It may not always be necessary to signal on the approach to the roundabout. You may not have to stop. If you do not have to stop, then look, listen carefully for traffic and continue as from point 3.

Note

For some mini-roundabouts you may need to signal on the approach and when you exit .

Remember your **'life-saver'** look.

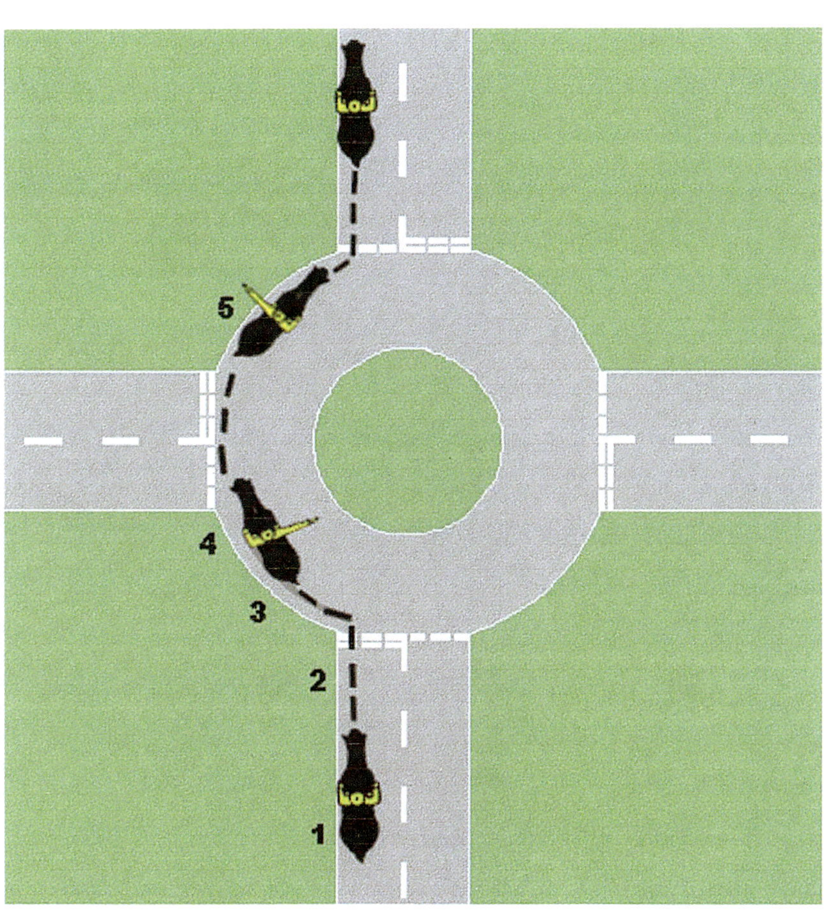

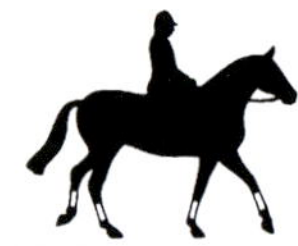

9. RIDING IN PAIRS AND RIDING IN GROUPS

Highway Code Rule 53

When riding on the road, you should never ride more than two abreast, and ride in single file on narrow or busy roads and when riding round bends.

The Department for Transport has confirmed that Rule 53 is not a legal requirement and it does not place any compulsion on riders to ride in single file. It provides general advice and guidance on safe riding, including where it may be advisable to ride in single file, but it remains the rider's decision whether or not they follow this advice according to particular circumstances. Rule 215 provides advice to other road users that they could encounter horse riders in double file in any circumstances, including when escorting a young or inexperienced horse or rider.

The distinction between legal requirements and advisory rules is made clear in the introduction to the Code, which can be viewed online at:

http://www.direct.gov.uk/en/TravelAndTransport/Highwaycode/DG 070236

Riding in pairs

- The more experienced rider/horse should be on the outside.
- Ride in single file where traffic and road conditions dictate.
- Do not obstruct other road users.
- Both riders should wear fluorescent, reflective clothing and both horses should wear fluorescent, reflective leg bands.
- Before setting out, explain the procedure for moving between single and double file and reasons for doing so.

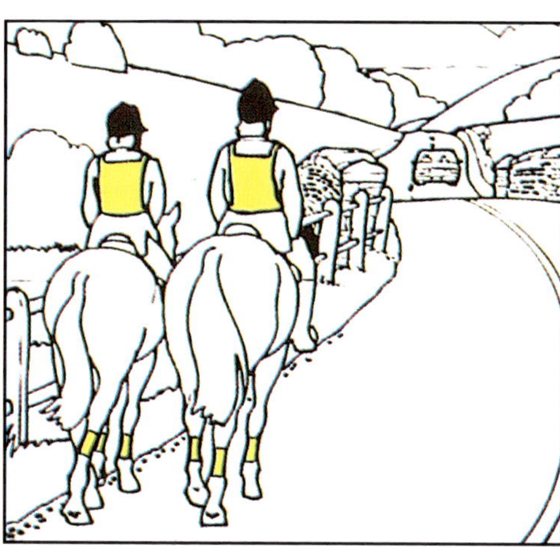

Two riders riding side by side approaching a narrow bridge. They see a car coming towards them.

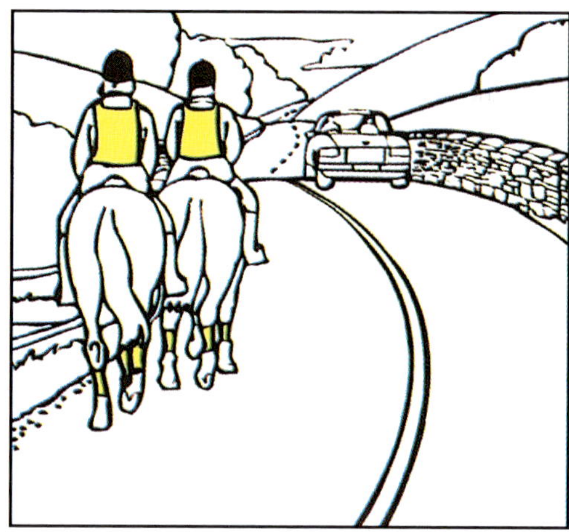

They move into single file to allow the car to pass.

Riding in a group

- All riders should wear fluorescent, reflective clothing.
- All horses should wear fluorescent, reflective leg bands.
- Where possible, place light-coloured horses on the outside as these will be more easily seen.
- Alert and sometimes defensive riding may be needed.
- Do not obstruct other road users.
- Do thank other road users who have been helpful.

How to ride as a group:

- Groups of riders should **not exceed eight**.
- Proceed in pairs. Leave a distance of **half a horse's length** between you and the horse and rider in front.
- Before setting out, explain the procedure for moving between single and double file and reasons for doing so.
  Take single file when necessary.
- The leader and last (rear rider) should give the signals and traffic communication. They should be in full control of the group. They should be mature and responsible.
- **Young, inexperienced horses and riders** should be placed **on the inside of the group**.
- Maintain a pace that is suitable for the whole group.
- Before departing, the plan of the ride and expected time of return should be given to a responsible person.

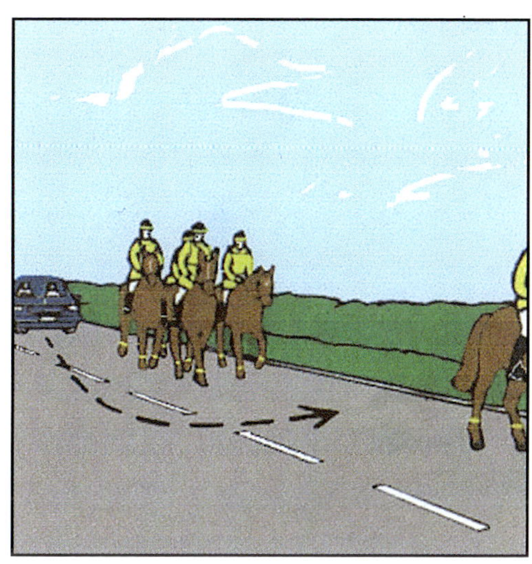

With large groups of riders e.g. sponsored rides, groups should be sub-divided, leaving a minimum of 30m between groups. This will enable traffic to overtake as safely as possible.

In some circumstances groups of riders from riding schools will find it more practical to remain as one group. If this is the case road junctions should be crossed as a single controlled group, monitored by the person in charge.

The ride leader should understand their legal and insurance responsibilities before escorting riders onto the public highway.

Be courteous, be responsible, be safe and be seen

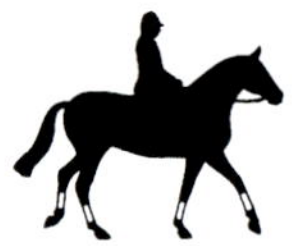

10. YOUNG RIDER, NOVICE RIDER, NOVICE HORSE

Novice or nervous horses

Highway Code Rules 52 and 215

Always ride with other, less nervous horses… Never ride a horse without both a saddle and bridle.

- Be particularly careful of horse riders… when overtaking. Always pass wide and slowly. …remember riders may ride in double file when escorting a young or inexperienced horse or rider…

A nervous or traffic-shy horse should only go out on the road in the company of an experienced horse. Avoid main roads and peak traffic times where possible.

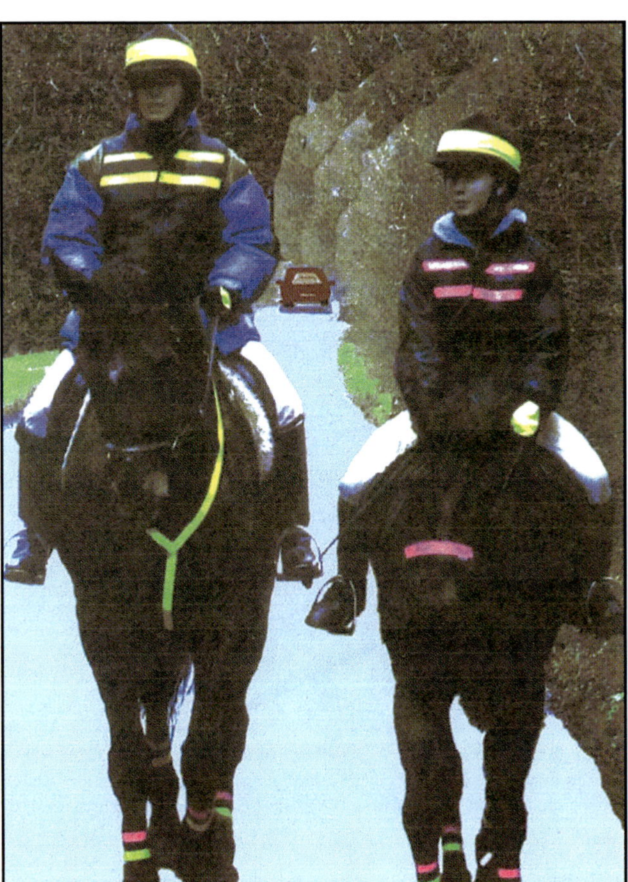

Novice riders

Highway Code Rule 52

- make sure you can control your horse.

Young riders

Highway Code Rule 49

- Children under the age of 14 MUST wear a helmet which complies with the regulations. It MUST be fastened securely.

Children cannot always judge the speed or distance of vehicles. Parents/guardians are responsible for deciding at what age their children may ride on public highways on their own.

Details of their intended route and estimated time of return should be left with a responsible person. This advice would apply to all riders.

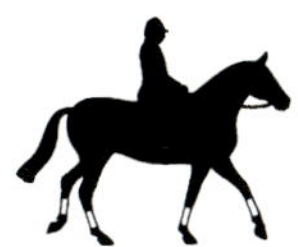

11. RIDING OR LEADING AFTER DARK, AT DUSK, OR IN INCLEMENT/DULL WEATHER

Highway Code Rule 51

- It is safer not to ride on the road at night or in poor visibility… A light which shows white to the front and red to the rear should be fitted with a band, to the rider's right arm and/or leg/riding boot.

Riding in these conditions should be avoided where possible. However if you must, make sure:

- you are wearing **reflective clothing** and your horse is wearing **reflective leg bands** fitted above the fetlock joints, preferably on all four legs.
- **You wear a light** showing white to the front and red to the rear.
- **When riding in a group**, the leading rider and the last (rear) outside rider should wear a light showing white to the front and red to the rear.

Understanding the difference between **reflective** and **fluorescent** material:

- **Fluorescent materials** show up in daylight but have no special qualities at night.
- **Reflective materials return (reflect)** a light source, either in daylight or darkness.

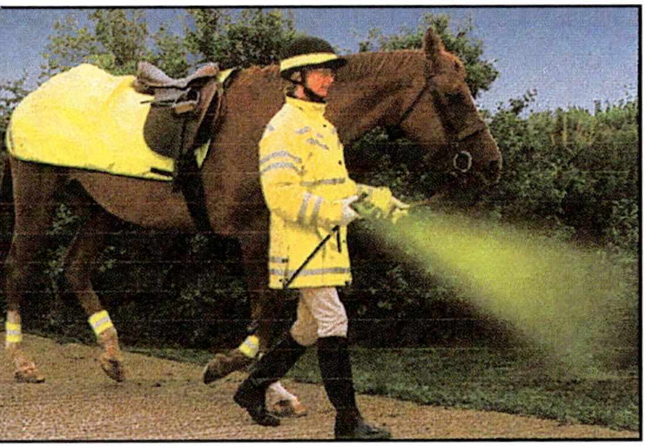

!

Fluorescent by day.

Reflective by night (can be worn day or night).

Highway Code Rules 51 and 53

- If you are leading a horse at night, carry a light in your right hand, showing white to the front and red to the rear…
- keep a horse you are leading to your left.

Leading a horse on foot

On the public highway keep to the left, **place yourself between your horse and the traffic** and ensure that both you and your horse are wearing reflective and fluorescent clothing with legs bands for your horse.

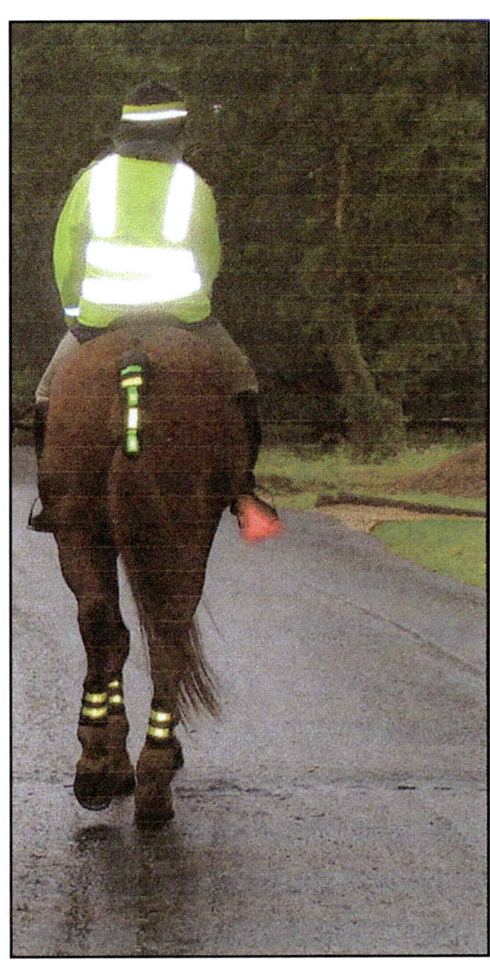

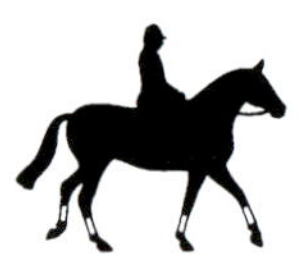

12. GRASS VERGES AND FOOTWAYS, BRIDGES AND UNDERPASSES

Grass verges and footways

> **Highway Code Rule 54**
> - You MUST NOT take a horse onto a foot path or pavement and you should not take a horse onto a cycle track. Use a bridleway where possible…

Where riding on verges is allowed, be aware of possible hazards, which may include rubbish, bottles and inspection hatches which may not be immediately apparent.

Cycle lanes

The Highway Code is unclear on the use of cycle lanes for horse riders. Common sense should prevail, but riders are warned that it is an offence to use cycle lanes where signs clearly indicate that horse riders are prohibited.

Railway bridges

- Look, check the traffic situation.
- Stop in good time if necessary.
- Never ride under a bridge if you hear a train approaching.

Bridges and underpasses

Wait for pedestrians to cross first when negotiating bridges and underpasses.
In some cases there is restricted headroom, if in doubt dismount and lead.

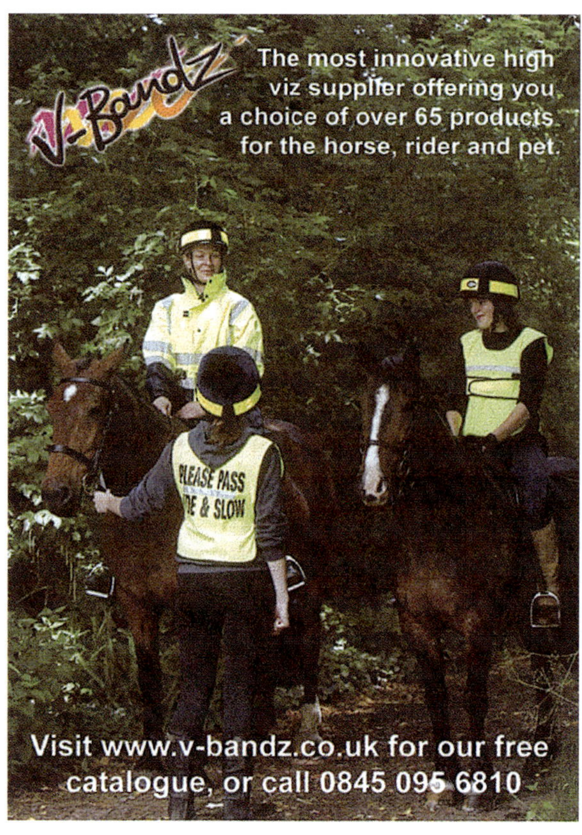

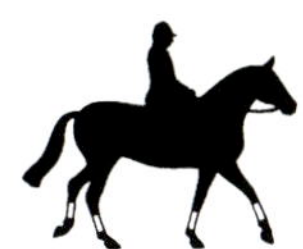

13. DANGEROUS ROAD CONDITIONS, WEATHER CONDITIONS AND EMERGENCY VEHICLES

Dangerous road conditions

- Worn, shiny patches on the road.
- Adverse camber especially on corners.
- Plastic paint (white lines, crossings, road markings) particularly when wet.
- Potholes and inspection covers.
- Loose grit and wet leaves.

Purpose made anti-slip studs, nails and horse-shoes can provide additional grip.

Snow and ice

You should not take your horse out on the public highway in these dangerous conditions. If you have reason to do so, keep your horse at a walk and do not hurry or have too tight a rein contact.

- Ride as near to the kerb or edge as is safe. The accumulation of grit will provide a better footing.
- Keep a rein contact with the horse at all times.
- Consider removing your feet from the stirrups.
- If the horse should slip and fall do not panic Keep calm; allow the horse to regain his footing. Check for injury.
- Move off the icy road before remounting.
- When riding in snow, smear grease thickly on the inside of the horse's feet.
- When leading a horse on foot, the horse should go at his own pace and you should concentrate on your footing.

Fog and mist

If caught in fog or mist take the same actions and precautions as you would when riding at dusk or at night.

Think ahead, be prepared

Windy weather

Highway Code Rules:227 and 232
- take extra care around pedestrians, cyclists, motorcyclists and horse riders
- gusts can also blow a car, cyclist, motor cyclist or horse rider off course...

- It will be harder to listen for other traffic.
- Horses will become tense and may be inclined to turn their quarters towards the wind. This could be into the traffic.
- You need to beware of plastic bags, flapping plastic in the hedges, silage bags, rattling gates and signs and rubbish on the public highway.

Emergency vehicles, incident support vehicles, agricultural vehicles and council vehicles

Take extra care if you hear the sirens of emergency vehicles or see their flashing lights. Both sirens and flashing lights have the potential to upset your horse. Many agricultural vehicles use flashing amber lights. Take an alternative route if possible.
Be careful at junctions especially those controlled by traffic lights. Approaching emergency vehicles may well pass through red lights.
It may be necessary to move to the side out of the way.

Look and listen

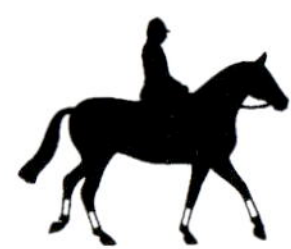

14. FALLS AND INJURIES

Unfortunately, even experienced riders may be thrown from a startled or frightened horse. It would be natural to panic in such a situation. Knowledge of what action to take should you be involved with an accident will help minimise the risk of further harm.

- Make safe.
- **Send someone** to warn traffic to slow down.
- The safety of the injured rider is most important, but If the horse or pony is loose, then send someone to try and catch it. Do not take risks or endanger the lives of others.
- **Ask for help** to call the appropriate emergency services as soon as possible. You will need to tell them the exact location.
- **Do not** remove the rider's hat.
- **Reassure the casualty** and stay with them. Try to keep them warm but try to avoid unnecessary movement.
- **Do not** put yourself or others at risk.
- **If necessary, and trained, start applying** the **ABC** of Emergency Aid. **Airway, Breathing, Circulation**.

Remember your safety and that of others is of paramount importance. Do not take risks

For further information, please refer to the current edition of the First Aid Manual, and section 7 (First Aid on the road) of the Annexes in the current edition of The Official Highway Code.

Accident Report Forms can be obtained from The British Horse Society, or downloaded from The BHS website. Please use these forms should you have an accident or a near miss. These reports contribute to campaigns for future safety improvements.

Have you remembered your insurance?

As a Gold Member of The British Horse Society free public liability insurance is automatically extended to you.

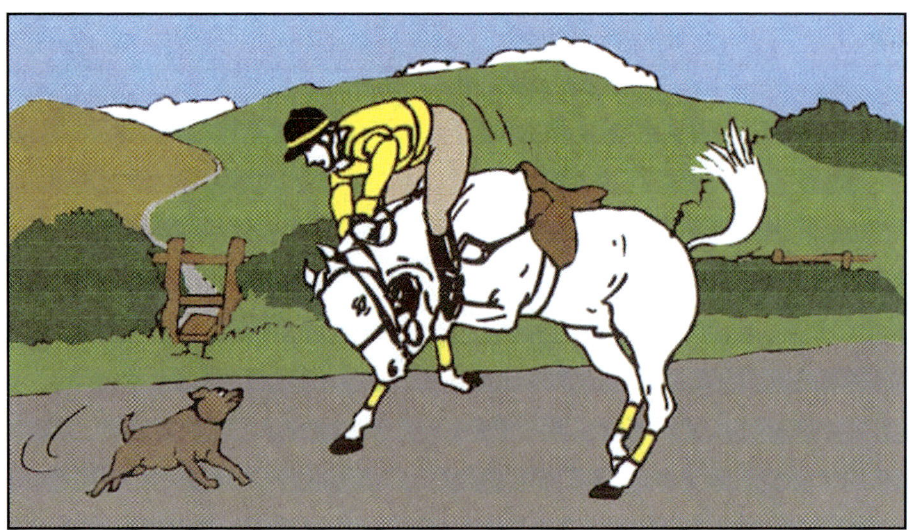

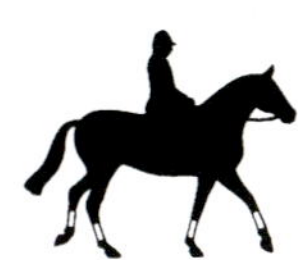

15. DRIVING HORSE-DRAWN VEHICLES

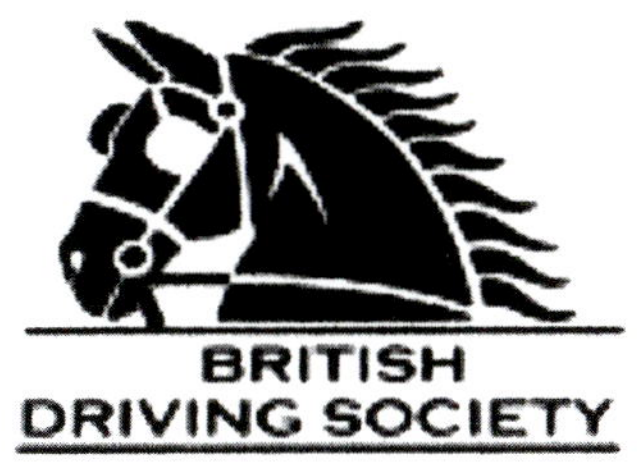

It is important that these guidelines are read in conjunction with the Official Highway Code, The British Driving Society's Guidelines on Road Safety for Harness Horse Drivers, the Introduction to Driving and the Department of Transport publication Code of Practice for Horse Drawn Vehicles. The BDS has its own Road Driving Assessment Test, details available from:

www.britishdrivingsociety.co.uk
Tel: 01437 892 001

Before going on the road

- Not only the harness, but also the vehicle's brakes, if any, wheels and shafts should be carefully checked. Brakes are not mandatory on horse drawn vehicles, but if fitted, they must be in working order. The whole vehicle should be in good working order before being driven on, or off, the road. Two wheeled vehicles should be correctly balanced.
- The horse/s must be sound and the feet well-shod.
- Attention must be paid to the welfare, safety and comfort of the horse. The harness and vehicle must fit the horse/s.
- Check that you are carrying the necessary spares. Carry a mobile phone so that you can summon help in an emergency.
- **Be safe, be seen**, rear reflectors must be fitted on modern vehicles, and lamps fitted and lit when driving after lighting-up time. Lamps need not be fitted nor lit if driving between the hours of dawn and dusk.
- You are advised to use reflective/fluorescent tabards and equipment for your horse, harness and vehicle.
- **Do not drive** on the road until you know that you can control your horse.

Arm signals

- You **must** know how to make the correct signals. They should be clear and positive.
- Try to establish eye contact with other road users.
- If the driver is unable to make the signals then the Assistant should make them. **Ensure** that your Assistant knows how to signal before going onto the road.
- For the **right turn** or move to the right the whip is kept under the left thumb and the arm held out the right as indicated above.
- For the **left turn** it is recommended your assistant signals with the left arm to the left.
- By holding the reins in the left hand, the right hand is free to support the left hand in order to maintain correct control of the horse and to carry the whip and make the signals.
- Remember **observe – signal – observe – manoeuvre**.

No signal exists if it has not been seen

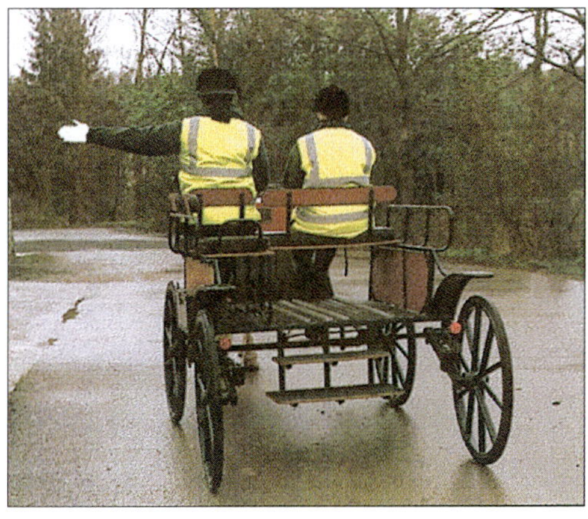

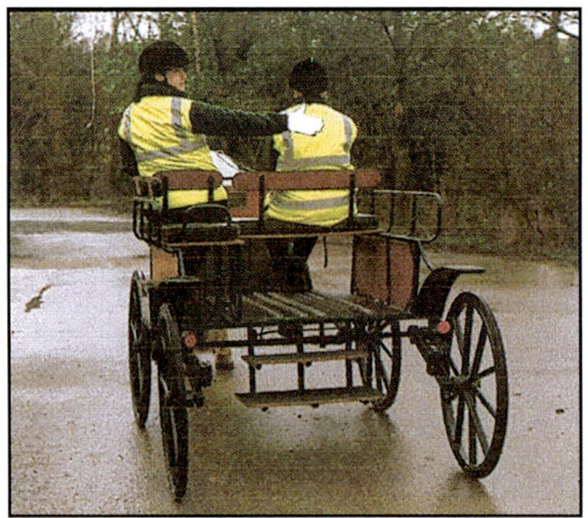

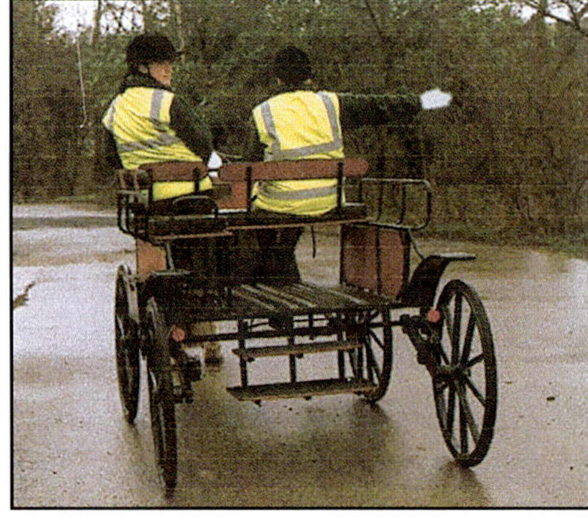

On the road

- You are strongly advised to have an **active assistant or passenger**, who can alight before blind bends and junctions and walk ahead to check that it is safe to proceed.
- If there is any doubt as to whether your horse will stand still at any place where you have to stop, **ask your assistant to dismount and hold the horse's head**.
- Train your horse to be confident in traffic by riding or leading him on the road in the company of an experienced horse, or long-rein him with a competent assistant. Avoid peak traffic times.
- **Slow down** and be careful and considerate when passing pedestrians, horse riders and other horse drawn vehicles.
- Thank other road users for their consideration, or ask your assistant to do so on your behalf. If you do not wish to take your hand off the reins then a nod and a smile is appropriate.
- When overtaking stationary obstacles only pass when it is safe to do so.
- Use your voice to communicate effectively with your horse.
- **Continually assess** the conditions and drive appropriately.
- Drive an even course near the left hand kerb. A wide gap may tempt a cyclist or motor cyclist to overtake on the near (left) side.

For future information please refer to the current National Occupational Standards Workbook Chapter on driving.

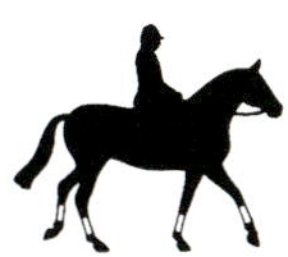

16. SIDE-SADDLE HORSE AND RIDER

Horse and equipment

The horse must be used to carrying a side-saddle, and must answer to the rigid whip.

The saddle must be in good condition and the tree must be sound. Special attention must be paid to the fixed pommel and the leaping head.

Buckles, girths and stitching must be in good repair.

The fit at the wither, shoulder and spine is important, with no pinching.

The seat should be level front to back. Packing on the near-side rear-panel must be greater than that on the off-side, *to allow the seat to sit level from side to side when the rider is in position*.

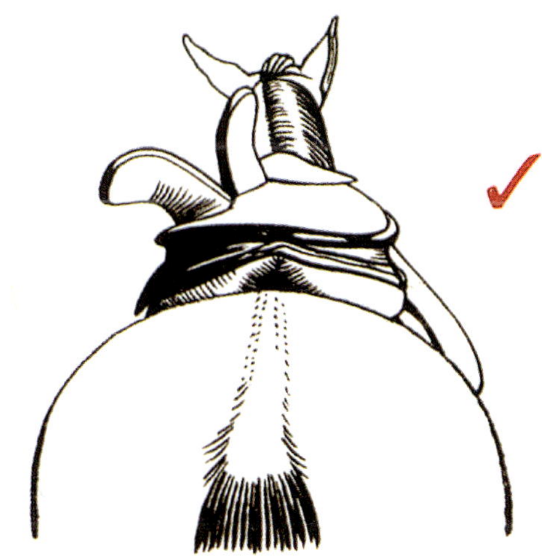

Saddle correctly fitted

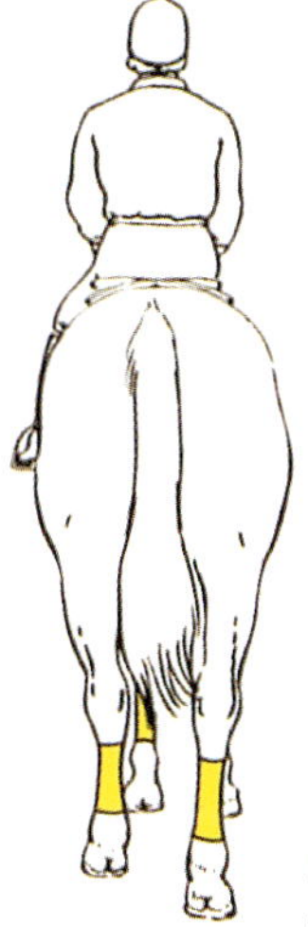

Rider sitting square, seat level from side to side

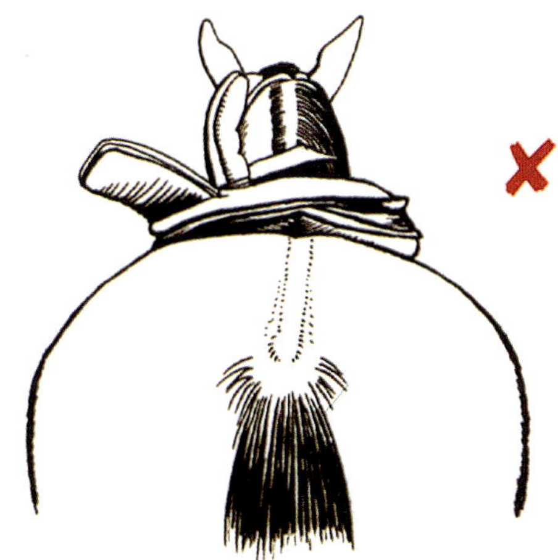

Saddle tilting left

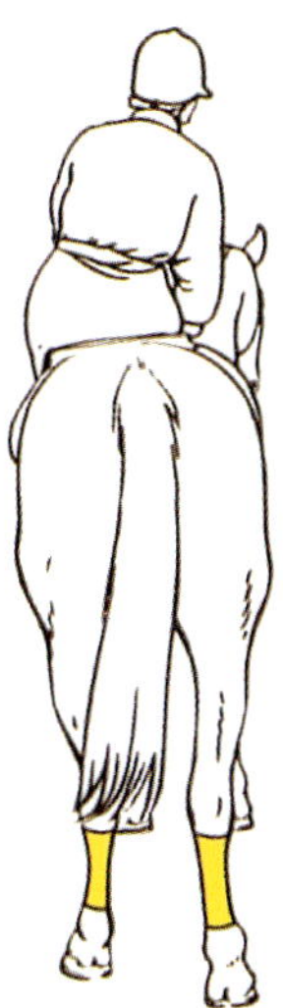

Insufficient packing on both sides, especially near side

Ideally the girth should be made of leather, and either plain or three-fold. It should be smooth, with a central keeper to accommodate a full-length balance strap and flap strap. The balance strap must be used.

Stirrup attachment – the safety fitting on the saddle and at the top of the stirrup leather must be in accord with the make of saddle.

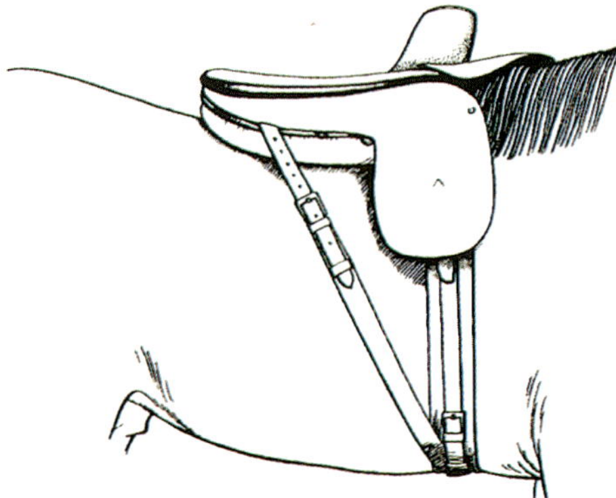

Position of balance strap in relation to girth

The stirrup iron must be 12mm (1½ inch) wider than the rider's boot. It should be in good condition and preferably of stainless-steel. If a roller bar is fitted to the saddle, the stirrup iron must be a safety-release type.

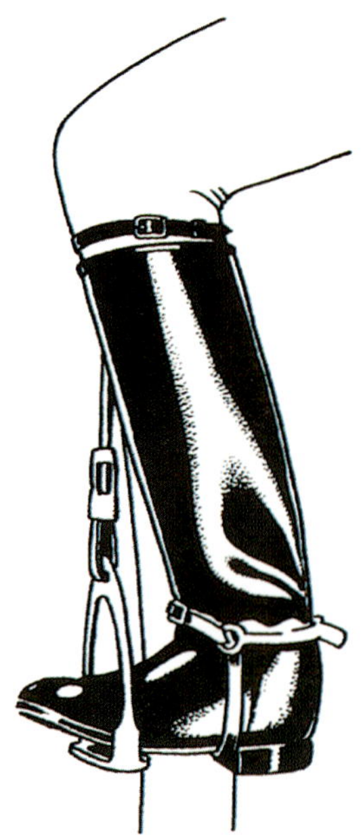

Leatherguard must cover billet hook. Note correctly fitted spur

Rider

A side-saddle habit need not be worn.

The rider's hat must conform to BS EN 1384 (97) or PAS 015 (94) or ASTM F1163.

A whip or rigid cane must be carried, a maximum length of 1m (39 inches), for use as a right leg aid.

A spur or spur-band may be worn by adult riders.

Note: Gloves should be light coloured to aid clarity of signals.

For advice on fit and condition of side-saddles, contact the local SSA Area Chairman or an instructor from the SSA Panel.

Side-saddle riders must be competent riding side-saddle, and be able to control their horse in walk, trot and canter. They must understand and be able to use the rigid whip to the correct effect.

To maintain control of the horse's quarters and ensure clear visibility over the right shoulder, side-saddle riders can approach hazards and junctions in a shallow 'shoulder fore' to the right.

There are no special concessions for side-saddle riders, in either control of the horse or safety.

Side-saddle riders should mention in their test application form that they will be riding side-saddle. This enables an appropriate examiner to be allocated.

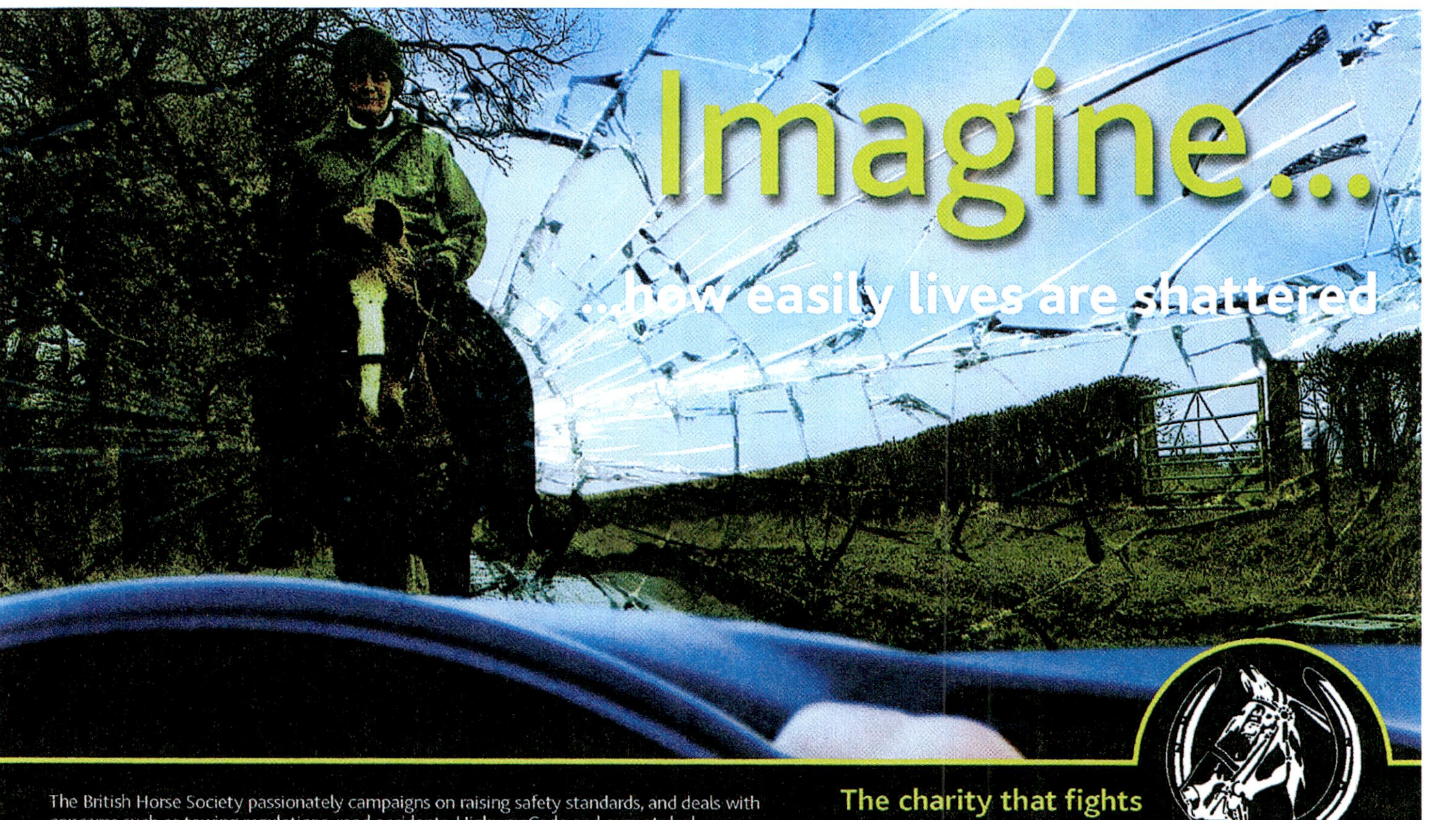
Imagine...
...how easily lives are shattered
The British Horse Society passionately campaigns on raising safety standards, and deals with concerns such as towing regulations, road accidents, Highway Code and a great deal more – all very real issues that could save your life from being shattered, or that of someone you know.
The Charity's Riding and Road Safety Test has the potential to save not only the rider's life, but that of their horse and other road users as well. Have you taken your BHS Riding and Road Safety Test?
To continue this vital work we need to recruit more members, after all, there's always more safety in numbers – so please join today.
The charity that fights on your behalf.
Join us now
The British Horse Society
call 08450 777728 or visit www.bhs.org.uk
Insurance • Welfare • Safety • Training • Exams • Approvals • Member benefits

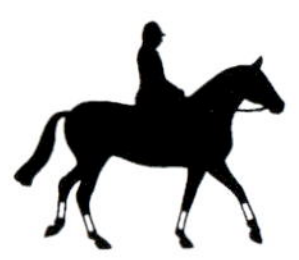

17. THE BHS RIDING AND ROAD SAFETY TEST

The aim

The aim of the test is to give recognition to responsible, courteous and competent riders well versed in road skills and road safety as set out within this Manual, the current edition of The Official Highway Code and the interactive training cd-rom.

Riding ability – All potential candidates for this test must be capable of riding independently at walk, trot and canter.

Whilst not compulsory, it is strongly recommended that riders have a minimum of 8-10 hours tuition from a BHS Approved Safety Trainer before they undertake this test.

The Test

Candidates will as a group, prior to the test, walk both the simulated and road routes with an examiner.

There will be a tack and turn-out inspection. This is to make sure that the horse's hooves/shoes, tack and the rider's clothing are in a safe and satisfactory condition. The rider's hat must be to the current standards and must be properly secured.

The test is divided into three sections:

SECTION 1: Theory Test

This is designed to test a rider's knowledge of The Highway Code, the meaning of traffic signals and the generally accepted rules for riding on the highway as set out within this Manual. Questions may be given orally or in the form of a written paper. This question paper is issued by the Safety Department. Each candidate will be given ten multi-choice questions to answer and a minimum score of **8 out of 10 (80%) must be achieved in order to move forward to Section 2**.

The theory section of the test may, in certain circumstances, be held on a day prior to the practical parts of the test.

SECTION 2: Simulated Road Test

This is designed to test, in an enclosed, controlled, safe, simulated road situation, a rider's precautions against - and reactions to – a series of noises and sights which might reasonably be met on the road, and which might cause a horse to shy. This will include road junctions, signs and traffic lights to test the candidate's ability to demonstrate control, road skills and their ability to use arm signals. Riders are also required to dismount and lead and remount. **A trot must also be shown during this part of the test. A minimum of 26 compulsory elements and 12 supporting elements must be achieved in order to move forward to Section 3**.

SECTION 3: Road Test

This is carried out on a planned risk-assessed, public road route. It is designed to test rider's road skills, road awareness, knowledge and application of the requirements of The Highway Code and of this Manual, in all genuine road situations. A trot should be shown during the test. **A minimum of 11 compulsory and 3 supporting elements must be achieved in order to complete the test successfully**.

A Local Authority Road Safety Officer or Police Officer may be invited to attend the test.

For riders riding side-saddle a Side-Saddle Association 'A' panel instructor will be invited to attend. Candidates must show their intention to ride side-saddle on their test booking form.

Note: the minimum age for candidates is twelve. The maximum age is seventy, unless that person has their own insurance. Horses and ponies must be five years old or over.

How do I apply for the Riding and Road Safety Test?

1. You can visit The BHS Safety website or you can contact The BHS Safety Department **(01926 707782)** you can also contact your local BHS Riding and Road Safety Representative (the details of which appear in *The BHS Yearbook*). They will be able to give you details of forthcoming tests in your area.
2. Application forms can be downloaded from the website. Application forms must be sent to the Safety Department along with the appropriate fee to arrive no later than 21 days prior to the test. Applications received 6 to 20 days prior to the test may be accepted subject to space being available on the test and subject to late payment fee. No applications are accepted within five working days of the test, this does not include the test day itself.

3. If you do not own a horse the Safety Department will be able to give you details of Road Safety Approved centres where you may hire a horse and do the test.
4. If you know of others who wish to take the test **(minimum of eight candidates)** it may be possible for examiners (and trainers) to come to you. This is subject to a Risk Assessment of the site and suitable road route (a fee is payable for this). Your County Road Safety representative will help you with this.

How can I organise some training and what aids are available to help me?

1. Whilst training is not compulsory, The BHS recommends a minimum of 8–10 hours tuition with a BHS Approved Safety Trainer. Details of Approved Safety Trainers may be found on The BHS Safety website or through your local representative and through The BHS Safety Department.
2. The Official Highway Code should be read in conjunction with the current edition of this book. Both are available through The BHS Bookshop.
3. You can download the Riding and Road Safety Syllabus from The BHS website.

Will I require any special clothing, equipment or fluorescent/reflective accessories?

You must have:

1. **A hat that conforms to the current recognised standards. The hat should be the rider's own hat, correctly fitted and secured with a minimum three point harness.**
2. **Boots or shoes with through soles.**
3. **Long sleeved clothing.**
4. **Gloves (dark coloured gloves are not permitted).**
   - **It is recommended that you carry a whip.**
   - **A fluorescent tabard will be provided for the test.**

Your horse must have:

1. **Correctly fitted supple tack.**
2. **Hooves and shoes that are in good condition.**
3. **Fluorescent leg bands are compulsory on both ridden sections of the test. These should be fitted on all four legs above the fetlock joints.**

Successful candidates will receive their certificates and badges direct from the Safety Department. Certification will be recorded. (A charge will be made for replacement certificates.)

Riding and Road Safety Syllabus

KEY: Assess during: T = Theory S = Simulated road route R = Road Test

Theory Section = 80% pass mark must be attained to move onto the simulated road route section. The question papers are made up of 10 questions taken from elements showing a T in the 'Assess during' column. Eight of the 10 questions must be answered correctly in order to move forward to the simulated road route section.

Simulated Road Route Section = 26 compulsory elements, all must be attained plus 12 supporting in order to move onto the road test.

This section requires the candidate to ride alone around a prescribed simulated road route in an enclosed area, addressing similar hazards and situations that they may encounter when riding on the public highway. Candidates need to demonstrate their understanding and ability to ride safely and responsibly.

Road Test = 11 compulsory elements must be attained plus 3 supporting in order to attain the BHS Level 2 Riding & Road Safety Test.

This section requires the candidate to ride alone around a risk assessed route on the public highway and demonstrate their ability to ride safely and responsibly.

Elements marked * indicate elements which could be covered in more than one section of the test. For instance in the theory section, the candidate could be asked to identify how they would ride around a corner (3.13.5*), where they will be expected to demonstrate how they would ride around a corner on the simulated road section (3.13.5*).

The candidate should be able to:	Element	Assess during	The candidate has achieved this outcome because s/he can:	Influence
Know, basic consideration and courtesy, insurance, novice or nervous horses, novice and young riders, tack and equipment, clothing, hats and footwear, whip and spurs riding or leading after dark, at dusk in inclement/dull weather, fog and mist as required for riding and or leading on the road	1.1.1	T	Identify the courtesy to be paid when meeting walkers	
	1.1.2*	T	Identify the courtesy to be paid when meeting cyclists	
	1.1.2*	R	Demonstrate the courtesy to be paid when meeting cyclists	Supporting
	1.1.3*	T	Identify the courtesy to be paid when meeting motorists	
	1.1.3*	R	Demonstrate the courtesy to be paid when meeting motorists	Supporting
	1.1.4	T	Identify the courtesy to be paid when meeting other riders	
	1.2.1	T	Identify the minimum form of insurance that every rider should have	
	1.3.1	**S & R**	**Demonstrate control of the horse when riding**	**Compulsory**
	1.3.2	S & R	Demonstrate correct use of the reins and stirrups when riding	Supporting
	1.3.3	S & R	Demonstrate effective use of the reins and legs when riding	Supporting
	1.3.4	S & R	Demonstrate a secure riding position	Supporting
	1.4.1	T	Identify where novice horses/riders should be positioned in a group of riders	
	1.4.2	T	Identify procedures adopted when a horse/pony is young and nervous in traffic	
	1.5.1*	T	Identify ill fitting and inappropriate tack	
	1.5.1*	**S**	**Identify ill fitting and inappropriate tack**	**Compulsory**
	1.5.2*	T	Recognise worn/weak, unsafe stitching	
	1.5.2*	**S**	**Recognise worn/weak, unsafe stitching**	**Compulsory**
	1.5.3*	T	Identify appropriate size and material for bits and stirrups	
	1.5.3*	**S**	**Identify appropriate size and material for bits and stirrups**	**Compulsory**
	1.5.4*	T	Identify the correct safe tack used when leading a horse	
	1.5.4*	S	Demonstrate the correct safe tack used when leading a horse	Supporting
	1.6.1*	T	State hooves and shoes that are in good condition	
	1.6.1*	**S**	**Identify hooves and shoes that are in good condition**	**Compulsory**
	1.7.1	T	Identify the Kitemark found in recommended riding hats	
	1.7.2	T	State one BHS recommended hat standard number	

The candidate should be able to:	Element	Assess during	The candidate has achieved this outcome because s/he can:	Influence
	1.8.1*	T	Identify suitable footwear for wearing when riding	
	1.8.1*	**S**	**Demonstrate suitable footwear for wearing when riding**	**Compulsory**
	1.9.1*	T	List appropriate clothing, worn when riding or leading on the highway	
	1.9.1*	**S**	**Demonstrate appropriate clothing, worn when riding or leading on the highway**	**Compulsory**
	1.9.2*	T	Identify the type of gloves suitable for wearing when riding and/or leading	
	1.9.2*	S	Demonstrate the type of gloves suitable for wearing when riding and/or leading	Supporting
	1.10.1*	T	Identify the reasons for wearing fluorescent clothing even in bright daylight	
	1.10.1*	**S**	**Demonstrate the reasons for wearing fluorescent/reflective clothing even in bright daylight**	**Compulsory**
	1.10.2	T	Identify the difference between fluorescent and reflective clothing	
	1.11.1	T	Identify what to wear or carry when leading a horse on the road after dark,	
	1.11.2	T	Identify what kind of clothing is safest if they must ride at night or in murky weather	
	1.11.3	T	Identify which riders and horses should wear fluorescent and reflective clothing when riding in a group	
	1.12.1*	T	Identify and/or demonstrate what to do with a whip when signalling	
	1.12.1*	S & R	Demonstrate what to do with a whip when signalling	Supporting
	1.12.2*	T	Identify why, when leading on the road, the whip is carried in the right hand	
	1.12.2*	S & R	Demonstrate why, when leading on the road, the whip is carried in the right hand	Supporting
Know the Highway Code it's Statutory Rules for stopping distances, traffic light signals, flashing red lights, road markings across the carriageway, signals by authorised persons, traffic signs, grass verges and footpaths, as they apply to leading and riding on the highway	2.1.1	T	State examples of stopping distances as described in the Highway Code	
	2.1.2	T	Identify circumstances that may influence stopping distances	
	2.2.1*	T	State the meaning of a green light at traffic lights	
	2.2.1*	**S**	**Demonstrate the meaning of a green light at traffic lights**	**Compulsory**
	2.2.2*	T	Identify when to be prepared to move off at the correct stage of the traffic light sequence	
	2.2.2*	**S**	**Demonstrate when to be prepared to move off at the correct stage of the traffic light sequence**	**Compulsory**
	2.2.3*	T	Identify which light or lights follow amber on its own at traffic lights	
	2.2.3*	**S**	**Demonstrate understanding of traffic light sequence**	**Compulsory**
	2.2.4*	T	State what the colour amber on its own means at traffic lights	
	2.2.4*	**S**	**Demonstrate what the colour amber on its own means at traffic lights**	**Compulsory**
	2.3.1	T	Identify a rider's action at a train level crossing with no gates, when the amber lights show prior to flashing red lights.	
	2.3.2	T	Identify the correct procedure at a level crossing, when the barriers come down, with the lights flashing and bells ringing	
	2.4.1*	T	Identify main road markings across the carriageway as indicated in the Highway Code	
	2.4.1*	**S**	**Demonstrate understanding of main road markings across the carriageway as indicated in the Highway Code**	**Compulsory**
	2.5.1	T	Identify the 'stop' signal to traffic approaching from behind given by authorised persons	

The candidate should be able to:	Element	Assess during	The candidate has achieved this outcome because s/he can:	Influence
	2.5.2	T	Identify the 'stop' signal to traffic approaching from the front given by authorised persons	
	2.5.3	T	Identify the 'stop' signal to traffic approaching from both front and behind given by authorised persons	
	2.6.1	T	Identify common traffic signs giving orders	
	2.6.2	T	Identify common traffic signs giving positive instruction	
	2.6.3	T	Identify common traffic signs giving warning	
	2.7.1	T	Identify the guidelines for riding on verges and paths used by pedestrians, cyclists and horse riders.	
Know roadcraft; courtesy, road awareness, road positioning, rider's signals, other useful signals, positioning at road junctions, T-junctions, left turns, right turns, flared junctions, cross-roads, traffic lights, roundabouts, stationary vehicles, dangerous/ noisy/ frightening hazards, railway bridges bridges and underpasses, u-turns, dismounting, leading and remounting, T-junctions, leading when mounted, riding in pairs or groups, groups of riders from riding schools, dangerous road conditions and snow and ice,	**3.1.1**	**S & R**	**Demonstrate correct positioning of the horse/ pony on the road**	**Compulsory**
	3.1.2	**S & R**	**Demonstrate correct safe positioning at road junctions**	**Compulsory**
	3.2.1	**S & R**	**Demonstrate 'observe, signal, observe, manoeuvre' sequence for changes of direction etc.**	**Compulsory**
	3.2.2	**S & R**	**Demonstrate vigilant observation when crossing a road**	**Compulsory**
	3.2.3	S & R	Demonstrate correct safe routines when passing stationary vehicles	Supporting
	3.3.1	**S & R**	**Demonstrate correct safe signalling procedure for left turns**	**Compulsory**
	3.3.2	**S & R**	**Demonstrate correct safe signalling procedure for right turns**	**Compulsory**
	3.3.3	S & R	Demonstrate correct safe signalling procedure to ask a driver to slow down	Supporting
	3.3.4	S & R	Demonstrate correct safe signalling procedure to ask a driver to stop	Supporting
	3.4.1	**S & R**	**Demonstrate correct safe routines when turning left at a T-junction**	**Compulsory**
	3.4.2	**S & R**	**Demonstrate correct safe routines when turning right at a T-junction**	**Compulsory**
	3.4.3	**S & R**	**Demonstrate correct safe routines when turning left**	**Compulsory**
	3.4.4	**S & R**	**Demonstrate correct safe routines when turning right**	**Compulsory**
	3.4.5	S & R	Demonstrate correct safe routines when turning left at a flared junction	Supporting
	3.4.6	S & R	Demonstrate correct safe routines when turning right at a flared junction	Supporting
	3.4.7	S & R	Demonstrate correct safe routines when turning left at a cross roads	Supporting
	3.4.8	S & R	Demonstrate correct safe routines when turning right at a cross roads	Supporting
	3.5.1	S & R	Demonstrate correct safe routines when turning left at traffic lights	Supporting
	3.5.2	S & R	Demonstrate correct safe routines when turning right at traffic lights	Supporting
	3.5.3	S & R	Demonstrate correct safe routines when going straight across at traffic lights	Supporting
	3.6.1*	T	Identify correct safe routines when negotiating roundabouts	
	3.6.1*	S & R	Demonstrate correct safe routines when negotiating roundabouts	Supporting
	3.7.1	S & R	Demonstrate effective correct safe routines when negotiating hazards	Supporting
	3.7.2	S & R	Demonstrate appropriate action when a noisy machine/hazard is in use at the side of the road and your horse shows signs of resistance	Supporting
	3.7.3	T	Identify how a very windy day, may create exceptional hazards	
	3.8.1*	T	Identify correct safe routines when negotiating bridges and underpasses and u-turns	
	3.8.1*	S & R	Demonstrate correct safe routines when negotiating bridges and underpasses and u-turns	Supporting

The candidate should be able to:	Element	Assess during	The candidate has achieved this outcome because s/he can:	Influence
	3.9.1*	T	Identify the correct safe procedure when dismounting and preparing to lead a horse/ pony	
	3.9.1*	**S**	**Demonstrate the correct safe procedure when dismounting and preparing to lead a horse/ pony**	**Compulsory**
	3.10.1*	T	Identify the correct safe method of leading a horse/ pony on the highway	
	3.10.1*	S	Demonstrate the correct safe method of leading a horse/ pony on the highway	Supporting
	3.10.2*	T	Identify the correct safe method of leading a horse/ pony that is wearing a running martingale	
	3.10.2*	S	Demonstrate the correct safe method of leading a horse/ pony that is wearing a running martingale	Supporting
	3.10.3	T	Identify correct safe procedure when leading a horse on foot on an icy road	
	3.10.4*	T	Identify the correct safe procedure for remounting	
	3.10.4*	**S**	**Demonstrate the correct safe procedure for remounting**	**Compulsory**
	3.10.5	T	Identify the correct safe method of leading a horse/ pony when mounted	
	3.11.1	T	State the maximum number of riders recommended to form a group on the road	
	3.11.2	T	State ideal distances kept between horses when riding in a group on the road	
	3.11.3	T	State the recommended maximum number of riders who should proceed as a group on the road, when dealing with large parties of riders	
	3.11.4	T	Identify how a group of riders should cross a main road	
	3.11.5	T	Identify when a group of riders should plan for carrying out changes from double file (two abreast) to single file and back again	
	3.11.6	T	Identify how a number of riders should proceed if a road is narrow or has bends	
	3.12.1	T	Identify examples of the essential requirements of the ride leaders legal responsibilities, when groups of riders from a riding school go out for a hack	
	3.12.2	T	Identify the correct procedure for crossing a road with a large riding school party	
	3.13.1	T	Identify the action taken if their horse continually slips on an icy or slippery road	
	3.13.2	T	Identify the road surface that will provide a better footing in snowy or icy road conditions	
	3.13.3	T	Identify the safest thing for a rider to do if the roads are icy	
	3.13.4	T	Identify what to do to improve the horse's footing when riding in snow	
	3.13.5*	T	Identify the most important reason for walking the horse round a corner	
	3.13.5*	**S**	**Demonstrate the most important reason for walking the horse round a corner**	**Compulsory**
Knows appropriate procedures for falls and injuries	4.1.1	T	Identify appropriate immediate action taken to secure the scene of an accident	
	4.1.2	T	Identify the ensuing action after securing the scene of an accident	
	4.2.1	T	State which area of the horses is struck in most road accidents	
	4.3.1	T	Identify the reasons for leaving a rider's hat on after a fall	
	4.4.1	T	Identify the ABC of emergency aid	
	4.5.1	T	Identify emergency action to stop bleeding	

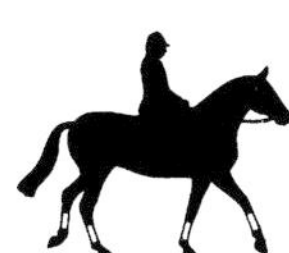

18. SAMPLE THEORY QUESTIONS

The traffic signs used on the following pages are © Crown copyright

1. If the roads are icy, what is the safest thing for a rider to do?
   a. **Ride the horse with a tight rein.**
   b. **Shorten the stirrup leathers.**
   c. **Not ride at all.**

2. At a level crossing, the barriers came down, with the lights flashing and bells ringing. What should you do?
   a. **Cross as quickly as possible.**
   b. **Stop in good time before the barrier.**
   c. **Dismount.**

3. You have a young/nervous horse, unused to traffic. Would you take him out on the road alone?
   a. **Yes, he must learn to be bold.**
   b. **No, go out in company to build his confidence.**
   c. **No, never take him out of the manege.**

4. A rider complains of a head injury after falling off her horse, should you?
   a. **Remove the hat and inspect the head injury.**
   b. **Leave the hat and wait for professional/ skilled medical help to arrive.**
   c. **Wait until the rider is able to stand up, then remount and ride home.**

5. Why should you look over your left shoulder before you turn left at a junction?
   a. **You should not.**
   b. **To check for cyclists.**
   c. **To make sure your horse's hindquarters are not pointing to the middle of the road.**

6. What is the difference between fluorescent and reflective clothing?
   a. **There is no difference.**
   b. **Fluorescent clothing is used in the dark, reflective clothing is used in bright daylight.**
   c. **Fluorescent clothing is used in bright daylight, and reflective clothing is used in the dark, and in dull conditions.**

7. If on a bridleway you meet pedestrians coming towards you, how would you pass them?
   a. **Walk past slowly and acknowledge them.**
   b. **Dismount and lead your horse past.**
   c. **Ignore them.**

8. According to the Highway Code, if a vehicle flashes its lights at you, what does it mean?
   a. **You may proceed.**
   b. **I am waiting for you.**
   c. **I am here.**

9. At traffic lights, what does the colour amber on its own mean?
   a. **Get ready to stop.**
   b. **Get ready to go.**
   c. **Stop.**

10. What is the minimum form of insurance that every rider should have?
    a. **Fire and theft.**
    b. **Personal accident.**
    c. **Personal liability.**

11. According to the Highway Code, are you allowed to ride or lead a horse or pony on a footpath or pavement?
    a. **Yes.**
    b. **No.**
    c. **Sometimes.**

12. When riding in a party divided into groups, what distances should there be between them?
    a. **30m (100ft).**
    b. **9m (30ft).**
    c. **15m (50ft).**

13. If you are going to collect your horse from the paddock and ride him home on the road, would you:
    a. **Take a headcollar?**
    b. **Take a saddle and bridle?**
    c. **Take a bridle?**

14. You are riding along a major road and wish to turn right into a minor road. A stream of traffic is approaching. Where would you stop and wait until the traffic had passed?
   a. **On the left of the major road, near the kerb or verge, opposite your new intended route.**
   b. **Just left of the centre line on the major road, opposite your intended route on the minor road.**
   c. **On the left of the major road, before the junction at the minor road.**

15. If a car in front of you has one or more white lights shining to the rear, which way would you expect it to move?
   a. **Forwards.**
   b. **Backwards.**
   c. **Turning.**

16. Nose rings are not to be worn when riding. What about earrings?
   a. **They should be removed.**
   b. **They may be worn**.
   c. **They may be worn only if they are studs.**

17. At traffic lights, what colour, or combination of colours, follows green?
   a. **Amber.**
   b. **Red and amber.**
   c. **Green and amber.**

18. When riding in a group on the road, what is the ideal distance that should be kept between horses?
   a. **Half a horse's length.**
   b. **A horse's length.**
   c. **Two horses' lengths.**

19. Describe the road sign for ROAD WORKS:
   a. **A rectangular, white background, red border, black silhouette of man shovelling grit.**
   b. **Triangular, white background, red border, black silhouette of man shovelling grit.**
   c. **Triangular, red background, white border, black silhouette of man shovelling grit.**

20. What is a rider required to do at a road junction where there is a continuous thick white line across the carriageway?
   a. **Stop at the STOP AND GIVE WAY sign.**
   b. **Give way to traffic on the major road.**
   c. **Stop and give way at the white line.**

21. Where should novice riders/horses be positioned in a group of riders?
   a. **On the outside to give the experience of traffic.**
   b. **On the inside, middle of the group.**
   c. **On the inside, at the front of the group.**

22. What is the first movement you should make before overtaking a parked vehicle or other obstruction?
   a. **Signal.**
   b. **Look all around.**
   c. **Change the whip to the inside hand.**

23. What is the correct sequence of traffic lights, starting from red?
   a. **Red.**
   b. **Amber.**
   c. **Red and amber.**
   d. **Green.**

24. According to the Highway Code, where must you never ride or lead a horse?
   a. **Footpath or pavement.**
   b. **Common land.**
   c. **In a one-way street.**

25. A rider SHOULD always wear a protective helmet to current standards. How should it be secured?
   a. **With a scarf.**
   b. **With a two-point harness.**
   c. **With a minimum three-point harness.**

26. What is the usual shape of road signs giving orders?
   a. **Circular.**
   b. **Triangular.**
   c. **Rectangular.**

27. How should a horse and rider negotiate a roundabout?
  a. **Choose the proper lane for the exit.**
  b. **Keep to the left.**
  c. **Horses and riders should never use roundabouts.**

28. If you are leading a horse either mounted or dismounted, where should you be positioned on the road?
  a. **On the left of the road, between the led horse and the traffic.**
  b. **Facing on-coming traffic, with you or the ridden horse nearest the verge.**
  c. **On the left with the led horse between you and the traffic.**

29. What is the procedure for crossing a main road when riding alone?
  a. **Look left, right, left again and cross quickly.**
  b. **Wait for a break in the traffic, then cross quickly.**
  c. **Look right, left, right again, behind and cross when the road is clear.**

30. Which insurance is automatically available to Gold Members of the British Horse Society?
  a. **Third party, fire and theft.**
  b. **Fully comprehensive.**
  c. **Third party legal liability.**

31. What is a rider required to do at a road junction where there is a double row of broken white lines across the carriageway?
  a. **Stop at the STOP AND GIVE WAY sign.**
  b. **Give way to traffic on the major road.**
  c. **Continue, as road signs do not affect riders.**

32. What shape is a road sign giving information?
  a. **Circular.**
  b. **Rectangular.**
  c. **Triangular.**

33. What does a green traffic light mean?
  a. **Go.**
  b. **Get ready to go.**
  c.. **Go only if it is safe to do so.**

34. If you can foresee a dangerous road hazard, what is the best action?
  a. **Ride on the pavement.**
  b. **Make the horse face up to it.**
  c. **Make a detour to avoid the hazard.**

35. When riding your horse/pony on the roads, are you required to obey all traffic signs and police signals?
  a. **Only those which relate to horse riders.**
  b. **All traffic signs and police signals must be obeyed.**
  c. **No, they do not relate to horse riders.**

36. If the road is icy, what precautions should a rider take?
  a. **Ride the horse with a tight rein.**
  b. **Quit the stirrup irons.**
  c. **Shorten the stirrup leathers.**

37. There is one eight-sided road sign – what does it tell you?
  a. **One-way street ahead.**
  b. **Roundabout ahead.**
  c. **Stop and give way.**

38. You are waiting to turn at a junction. A car on the major road is signalling to turn left into your road. Should you:
  a. **Carry on with your turn?**
  b. **Wait until the road is clear?**
  c. **Wave him on?**

39. What road marking would you expect to find when you have to give way to traffic when joining a major road?
  a. **Single broken white line across the carriageway.**
  b. **Single continuous white line across the carriageway.**
  c. **Double broken white lines across the carriageway.**

40. Triangular signs with white background, and red borders:
  a. **Give orders?**
  b. **Give information?**
  c. **Give warnings?**

41. What does the Highway Code direct that you must be able to do before riding your horse on the road?
  a. **Be used to riding in traffic.**
  b. **The horse is used to traffic.**
  c. **You can control your horse.**

42. According to the Highway Code, if you are riding a horse on the public highway after dark, what should wear?
a. **A flashing amber light.**
b. **A reflector on the back of your hard hat.**
c. **A light showing white to the front, red to the rear.**

43. At traffic lights, what colour follows amber on its own?
a. **Green.**
b. **Red.**
c. **Red and amber.**

44. A policeman or traffic warden on duty puts his hand up with the palm towards you, what must you do?
a. **Wave back.**
b. **Dismount.**
c. **Stop.**

45. When riding past a hazard on the side of the road, which is safest?
a. **Bend the horse's head towards the hazard.**
b. **Bend the horse's head away from the hazard.**
c. **Keep his head straight.**

46. What should a rider always carry in his pocket?
a. **Money/phone card or mobile phone.**
b. **String.**
c. **A folding hoof-pick.**
d. **All of the above.**

47. What is the principal reason why you, as a rider, should avoid trotting round corners/ bends in the road?
a. **To avoid tiring the horse.**
b. **The road surface may be very slippery.**
c. **To avoid stressing the horse's legs.**

48. How is a party of riders advised to cross a main road?
a. **Each rider to cross individually, each making his own judgment.**
b. **Cross in pairs, leading rider to make the decision when to cross.**
c. **Wait until all riders can cross the road together without leaving anyone behind.**

49. If on a bridlepath you meet pedestrians coming toward you, would you:
a. **Walk past slowly?**
b. **Dismount and lead your horse past?**
c. **Ignore them?**

50. How should a rider negotiate a roundabout?
a. **Choose the same lane as you would when driving a car.**
b. **Keep to the left.**
c. **Horses and riders should never use roundabouts.**

51. What position on the road would you adopt if you were taking the third exit at a roundabout?
a. **Cut across the central island.**
b. **On the right of the road.**
c. **On the left of the road.**

52. What is the most important item to check on the horse before going out on the road?
a. **His coat should gleam.**
b. **His shoes and hooves should be in good condition.**
c. **Hooves should be oiled.**

53. Tick three items of importance that the rider should wear:
a. **Protective helmet to current standards.**
b. **Tie.**
c. **Jodhpurs.**
d. **long-soled boots with a heel.**
e. **Hacking jacket.**
f. **Fluorescent/reflective tabard.**

54. Tick three items of importance for the horse to wear before going out on the road:
a. **Saddle.**
b. **Numnah.**
c. **Brushing boots.**
d. **Bridle.**
e. **Fluorescent/reflective leg bands.**
f. **Coloured browband.**

55. When would a group of riders ride in single file?
a. **On a major road.**
b. **Approaching a road junction.**
c. **Road narrows, or on approach to a bend.**

56. Which three of the following items does the Highway Code stipulate when riding at night on the road?
a. **Stirrup lamp.**
b. **Blinkers on the horse.**
c. **Torch.**
d. **Riding on verges.**
e. **Dismount and lead.**
f. **Reflective clothing.**
g. **Reflective leg bands.**

57. If you are riding a horse and leading another, the led horse should be on your:
a. **Left?**
b. **Right?**
c. **Behind you?**

58. If your horse continually slips on an icy or slippery road, what action should you take?
a. **Hope for the best.**
b. **Quit your irons and ride near to the verge/kerb.**
c. **Trot on to get clear of the problem as soon as possible**.

59. A party of thirty-two riders wish to proceed on the public highway. What is the maximum number who should proceed as a group on the road?
a. **The lot.**
b. **Groups of sixteen.**
c. **Groups of five.**
d. **Groups of eight.**

60. Which sign means 'One-way traffic'?

a. 

b. 

c. 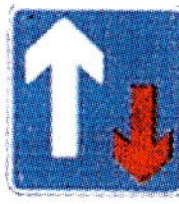

61. At a level crossing,the barriers come down, with the lights flashing and bells ringing. What should you do?
a. **Cross as quickly as possible.**
b. **Stop in good time before the barrier.**
c. **Dismount.**

62. You have a young/nervous horse, unused to traffic. Would you take him out alone?
a. **Yes, he must learn to be bold.**
b. **No, go out in company to build his confidence.**
c. **No, never take him out on the road.**

63. Where should as rider's hands be when overtaking an obstruction/hazard on the side to the road?
a. **On the reins.**
b. **Signalling.**
c. **Reins in one hand.**

64. If you keep your horse at grass a distance from home and you need a bucket of food with which to catch him, would you:
a. **Take the bucket and feed with you from home and ride back with the bucket on your arm?**
b. **Leave the bucket in the field?**
c. **Take the feed down in your pocket to catch your horse?**

65. What should you always do when a driver or other road user has been helpful and considerate to you as a rider|
a. **Ride on.**
b. **Get out of his way.**
c. **Acknowledge his courtesy with a nod and a smile.**

66. A very noisy machine is in use at the side of the road. What should you do?
a. **Keep going, urging your horse on.**
b. **Ask the operator to switch off the machine. Ride past thanking him.**
c. **Swith on your Walkman.**

67. Some train level crossings with no gates have amber lights followed by flashing red lights. When the amber lights are showing, should you:
a. **Hurry across before the train comes?**
b. **Wait until all the lights go out, then cross?**
c. **Consult a railway timetable?**

68. When riding behind a slow-moving car at the approach to a cross-roads, the driver makes an anti-clockwise circular movement with his right hand and arm. What is he signalling too the road users?
a. **You are to overtake him.**

b. **He is turning right.**
c. **He is turning left or pulling into the left.**

69. On which one of the following can you ride or lead?
a. **Motorway.**
b. **Footpath.**
c. **Bridleway.**

70. At a pelican crossing does flashing amber mean:
a. **Stop?**
b. **Move off?**
c. **Move off only if the crossing is clear of pedestrians?**

71. Which footwear is ideal for riding?
a. **Trainers.**
b. **Riding boots with through soles.**
c. **Wellingtons.**

72. Which of the following describes the sign for NO ENTRY:
a. **Horizontal red bar a white disc?**
b. **Horizontal white bar on a red disc?**
c. **Horizontal white bar on a blue disc?**

73. Which is the most important reason for walking your horse round a corner?
a. **In case you meet something.**
b. **To give your horse a chance to see where he is going.**
c. **Because the road surface is often slippery.**

74. Under legislation which has been in place since 1991, at what age are young people required to wear hard hats when riding on the road?
a. **Up to ten years.**
b. **Up to fourteen years.**
c. **Up to eighteen years.**

75. There is some headgear which is acceptable under the recent legislation concerning hard hats for young people when riding on the road but which is not acceptable to The British Horse Society. It is:
a. **Polo helmets?**
b. **Pedal cycle helmets?**
c. **Jockey skull caps?**

76. You are on your horse and waiting to turn right into a minor road from a major road. The headlights from an oncoming car flash twice. What does this mean according to the Highway Code?
a. **It doesn't mean anything.**
b. **Get out of my way.**
c. **I am here.**
d. **You may turn across.**

77. What is the meaning of this road sign?
a. **Series of bends.**
b. **Double bend.**
c. **Slip road to motorway.**

78. What is the meaning of this road sign?
a. **Footpath only.**
b. **Pedestrian crossing.**
c. **Footpath end.**

79. As a horse rider, how can you request a driver to stop?
a. **By calling out to him.**
b. **By holding your hand up, palm out.**
c. **By giving the slowing-down signal.**

80. What does this road marking mean?
a. **Parking zone.**
b. **Warning of 'Give Way' junction ahead.**
c. **Traffic island.**

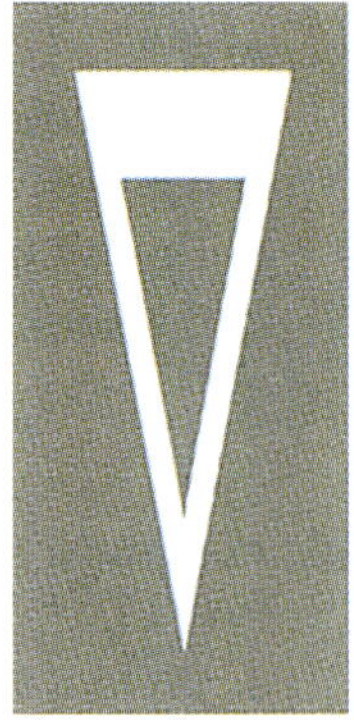

81. At a pelican crossing what colour light do you see, as a road user, when the green man is flashing for pedestrians?
a. **Red.**
b. **Flashing amber.**
c. **Green.**

82. What is the meaning of this road sign?
a. **Sharp deviation.**
b. **Petrol station ahead.**
c. **Count-down markers.**

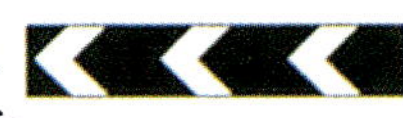

83. What does this signal, given by a police officer, mean?

a. **Stop, to traffic from the front.**
b. **Stop, to traffic from behind.**
c. **Stop, to traffic from the front and behind.**

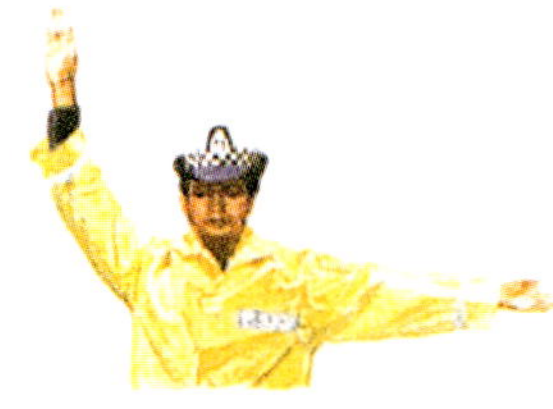

84. What is the meaning of this road marking?

a. **School, keep clear.**
b. **Do not enter the marked area unless your exit is clear or you are intending to turn right.**
c. **Superstore car parking ahead.**

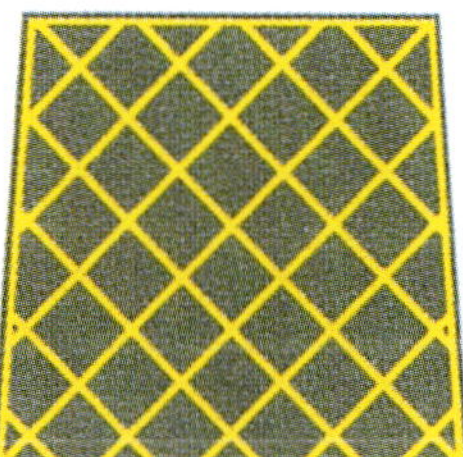

85. When you are riding along the highway, in which hand should you carry your whip?

a. **It depends whether you're left-handed or right-handed.**
b. **The left hand.**
c. **The right hand.**

86. As a horse rider, can you proceed past this road sign?

a. **On foot only.**
b. **Yes.**
c. **No.**

87. What does this road sign mean?

a. **Accident ahead.**
b. **Slippery road.**
c. **Beware of drunken drivers.**

88. Which of the following is not a current British Standard for protective headgear for horse riders?

a. **PAS 015 Kitemarked.**
b. **BS EN 1384 Kitemarked.**
c. **BS 6473 Kitemarked.**

89. What does this road marking mean?

a. **Give way to traffic on a major road.**
b. **Give way to pedestrians.**
c. **Stop until the green light shows.**

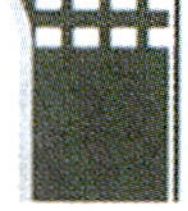

90. What is the meaning of this road sign?

a. **Level crossing without a barrier.**
b. **Cross roads ahead.**
c. **No waiting.**

91. What is the meaning of this road sign?

a. **T-junction.**
b. **dead end to the right.**
c. **No heavy goods vehicles.**

92. This road sign means that the national speed limit applies. What is the maximum national speed limit on a single carriageway road?

a. **80mph.**
b. **70mph.**
c. **60mph.**

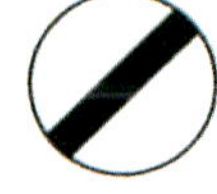

93. What is the meaning of this road sign?

a. **Pony Club camp.**
b. **Parking place.**
c. **Press entrance.**

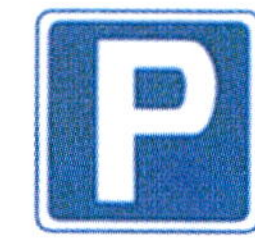

94. What is the meaning of this road sign?

a. **Gated level crossing.**
b. **Cattle market ahead.**
c. **School gates.**

95. Which of the following describes a hazard warning line?

a. **Short lines with long gaps.**
b. **Double white lines.**
c. **Long lines with short gaps.**

96. What do the zig-zag lines on the approach to a zebra crossing mean?

a. **Do not wait or park on the zig-zags.**
b. **Pedestrians may be crossing on the zig-zags.**
c. **Keep clear of lines when pedestrians are crossing.**

97. What is the meaning of this road sign?

a. **Slippery road.**
b. **Double bend.**
c. **Overhead electric cables.**

98. Which of the following statements is the law's demand?

a. **You must not ride a horse on the highway unless you have passed the Riding and Road Safety Test.**
b. **You must not wilfully ride a horse on the footpath.**
c. **You must not ride a horse under the age of four on public roads.**

99. What is the meaning of this road sign?

a. **Forestry Commission.**
b. **Christmas shoppers' parking.**
c. **Wild animals.**

100. It is estimated that eight road accidents involving horses occur each day in the UK. In almost fifty per cent of these accidents, horses are struck from:

a. **The rear?**
b. **The side?**
c. **The front?**

101. Which of these road signs means T-junction?

a. **b.** **c.**

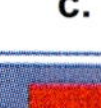

102. Which of these road signs warn of cattle?

a. **b.** **c.**

103. What does this road sign mean?

a. **Concealed entrance to driveway.**
b. **Level crossing without barrier.**
c. **Cross-roads ahead.**

104. What does this road sign mean?

a. **One-way traffic only.**
b. **Mini roundabout.**
c. **Turning area.**

105. What is the meaning of this road sign?

a. **No horse riding.**
b. **Horse riders only.**
c. **Accompanied horses**

106. What wording is missing from this road sign? Is it:

a. **NO ENTRY?**
b. **STOP?**
c. **ROUNDABOUT?**

107. Which of the following white lines would you see across the roadway if there is a GIVE WAY sign before a major road?

a.

b.

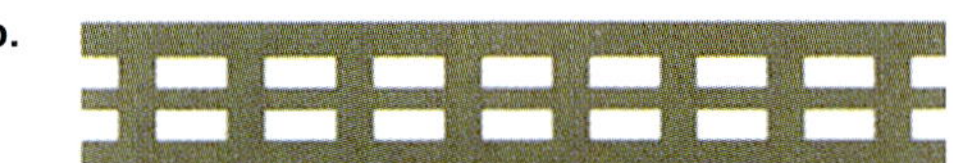

c.

108. Approximately how many road accidents involving horses occur annually in the UK, according to BHS estimates?

a. **800.**
b. **1250.**
c. **3000.**

109. What is the meaning of this road sign?

a. **Gas leak.**
b. **Other danger.**
c. **Overhead cable.**

110. What is the meaning of this road sign?

a. **T-junction.**
b. **No through road.**
c. **Traffic merges from the right.**

111. What does this driver's arm signal mean to you as a horse rider?

a. **You may overtake me.**
b. **I intend to move into the left or turn left.**
c. **I am going to slow down.**

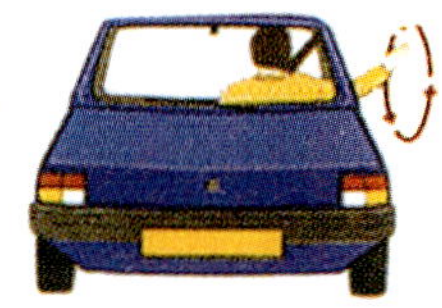

112. What is the meaning of this road sign?

a. **Loose chippings.**
b. **Beware! Landslide.**
c. **Excessive spray.**

113. What is the meaning of this road sign?

a. **Pass either side.**
b. **Keep left unless turning right.**
c. **Centre lane closed.**

Side-saddle candidates will receive additional sheets to include: positioning for maximum visibility on the road/at junctions/approaching hazards/dismount, leading and remount.

PUBLIC RIGHTS OF WAY

Horse riders and walkers have equal rights on bridleways; cyclists must give way to pedestrians and horse riders.

(Section 30, Countryside Act 1968)

All 'public rights of way' are highways in law and anyone may use them provided they keep to the line of the path and do not roam at will over the land. Some types have restrictions for use which must be obeyed. Generally speaking the highway authority is responsible for the maintenance of the surface of rights of way, and the landowner/ occupier is responsible for keeping passage clear from overhanging vegetation, crops etc.

Types of rights of way

Footpath – pedestrians only.

Bridleway – ridden or led horses, but not driven. Pedestrians and pedal cyclists also allowed.

Byway Open to All Traffic (BOAT) – also known simply as byway, can be used by all including horse-drawn vehicles or motor vehicles.

Restricted Byways (formerly RUPPs) – horse traffic, cyclists, walkers and any vehicle that is not mechanically propelled may use a restricted byway.

Maps

All rights of way are shown on the Definitive Map for any given area. This map is lodged in County Council offices and some District Council offices, and is available for the public to see; sometimes an appointment is necessary. It gives up-to-date information, as any changes to right of way are required to be made to it. You can check your own Ordnance Survey (OS) map against this map for accuracy.

A variety of Ordnance Survey (OS) Maps are available to cover the whole country; all show public rights of way. Landranger with a scale of 1:50,000 covers a large area but does not give so much detail. Most commonly used are the larger scaled (1:25,000) Outdoor Leisure, Pathfinder and Explorer maps. The Explorer maps are now gradually replacing Outdoor Leisure and have replaced the Pathfinders which are extinct from Summer 2003. The larger scale maps all show field boundaries.

Rights of way on maps

Rights of way are shown on maps by the following markings:

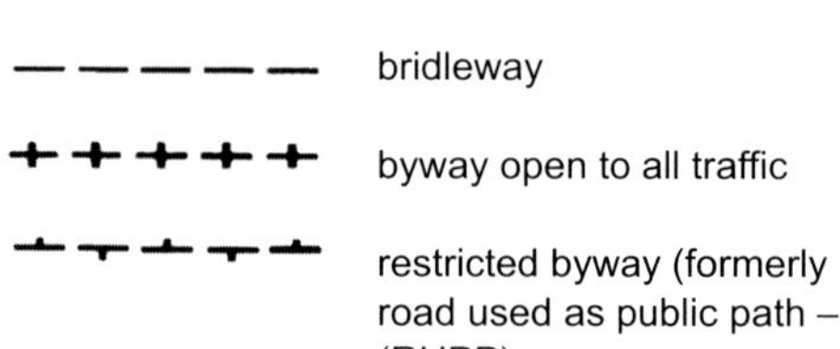

On 1:25,000 maps these markings are coloured green, whilst on 1:50,000 (Landrangers) they are shown in pink.

Waymarkers

A wide variety of waymarkers are used to show where a right of way leaves the road. They should also appear at strategic points along the way. The type of right of way is identified by a coloured arrow, i.e. yellow for footpath, blue for bridleway, and red for byway, pointing, as near as is practicable, in the direction of the route.

Other access routes

Canal and river towpaths. Legally, towpaths are for river users. Some have been dedicated as rights of way, but river users take precedence and you may find byelaws or other restrictions. Many do not allow horses at all on safety grounds, if only because of the narrow paths, lack of headroom on bridges and suitable access points.

Permissive paths (shown only on Explorer maps). These are paths that are not public rights of way, but which the landowner has agreed can be used by the public, with certain conditions. They are often waymarked in the same colours as public rights of way, but sometimes in white to emphasis their difference. You may also find permissive paths in open spaces such as country parks and common land. They are only occasionally shown on maps, in the same format as public rights of way but coloured red.

Many public open spaces carry their own codes or byelaws relating to riding and driving. Special maps are often available showing the riding tracks and horse rides, and other publications such as The British Horse Society's *On Horseback* series offer further choice.

PUBLIC RIGHTS OF WAY SAMPLE QUESTIONS

1. Where can't you legally ride?
   - **a.** Footpath.
   - **b.** Bridleway.
   - **c.** BOAT.
   - **d.** Restricted Byway.
   - **e.** Motorway.

2. Where will you find the Definitive Map?
   - **a.** Stationery shop.
   - **b.** Newsagents.
   - **c.** Council Offices.

3. Which type of Ordnance Survey map shows field boundaries?
   - **a.** Explorer.
   - **b.** Landranger.
   - **c.** Outdoor Leisure.

4. Which of the following markings does not give access to horses?
   - a. + + + + +
   - b. — — — — —
   - c. - - - - - - - - - - - -

5. What colour denotes a bridleway on a waymarker (it could be a post or a narrow)?
   - **a.** Blue.
   - **b.** Orange.
   - **c.** Yellow.

6. What is a permissive path?
   - **a.** A legal right of way.
   - **b.** A privately owned path with the landowner's permission for use.

7. If shown on an OS map, what colour markings will you see for a permissive path?
   - **a.** Green.
   - **b.** Black.
   - **c.** Brown/orange.

8. Who is responsible for maintaining the surface of public rights of way?
   - **a.** The local highway authority.
   - **b.** The landowner.
   - **c.** The users.

Recommended reading

BHS Access Leaflet:

Code for Riding and Driving Responsibly

Countryside Agency Publications:

Out in the Country

Horses in the Countryside

Waymarking Public Rights of Way

USEFUL INFORMATION

By visiting the BHS website www.bhs.org.uk these are some of the items you can download:

* A Membership Application Form
* Details of Riding and Road Safety Tests
* A Riding and Road Safety Test Application Form
* An Accident Report Form
* An Incident Report Form for Fireworks
* An Incident Report Form for Dog Attacks
* Guidlines for Highway Authorities on Horse and Highway Surfacing
* Ministry of Defence Safety Guides and Poster on Low Flying Helicopters

INDEX

Note: Page numbers in *italics* refer to sample theory questions

THE BRITISH HORSE SOCIETY

RIDING AND ROAD SAFETY TEST

APPLICATION AND ENROLMENT

This test is open to any rider between the ages of 12 and 70 years.
Up to date application forms are available on request from:

The Safety Department
The British Horse Society
Stoneleigh Deer Park
Kenilworth
Warwickshire
CV8 2XZ

or by telephoning: 0844 848 1666 or 01926 707700

Or by fax: 01926 707800

Or by email: enquiry@bhs.org.uk

Application forms must be submitted to the Safety Office
no later than 21 days before the date of your proposed test,
so please allow plenty of time for us to receive your application form.

Good luck, and safe riding!

Confidential
*Form **RS03***

THE BRITISH HORSE SOCIETY
ACCIDENT REPORT

By completing this form you will help in putting together much needed statistics on horse-related traffic accidents, of which there are at least eight each day. The figure may be greater than this. Your contribution to our statistics will help to improve on that situation.

If more than one horse or rider involved please complete a separate form for each and staple them together

Date of accident: day of week ☐ 1 date ☐☐ month ☐☐ 2 year ☐☐ 3

Time to the nearest hour: ☐ a.m. 4 or ☐ p.m.

Town/Village/District: ______________ **County:** ______________ 5

ENTER NUMBERS OF EACH TYPE OF ROAD USER INVOLVED IN APPROPRIATE BOXES:

6. Those involved:
horse ☐ 1 rider ☐ 2 pedestrian ☐ 3 pedal cycle ☐ 4 motor cycle ☐ 5 car/van ☐ 6 farm machinery ☐ 7
lorry ☐ 8 bus/coach ☐ 9 not known ☐ other ☐ 10 specify ______________

TICK ONLY ONE MOST APPROPRIATE BOX FOR EACH OF THE FOLLOWING QUESTIONS:

7. Was the horse:
ridden ☐ 1 led by walker ☐ 2 led by rider ☐ 3 loose ☐ 4 in harness ☐ 5 not known ☐
other ☐ 6 specify ______________

8. Was the rider:
alone ☐ 1 with one other horse ☐ 2 wih a group of horses (more than 2) ☐ 3 not known ☐ no rider involved ☐ 4 *(if no rider involved go to question 16)*

9. Was rider wearing a hard hat:
no ☐ 1 yes ☐ 2 not known ☐ *(if rider was not wearing a hard hat go to question 13)*

10. Was hat displaced during the accident:
no ☐ 1 yes ☐ 2 not known ☐

11. Was the hat:
EN 3184 ☐ 1 PAS 015 ☐ 2 ASTM F1163 ☐ 3 not known ☐ other ☐ 5 specify ______________

12. How was the hat secured:

no strap/ harness	elastic strap	simple chinstrap	harness	harness & chinstrap	not known
☐ 1	☐ 2	☐ 3	☐ 4	☐ 5	☐

other ☐ 7 specify ______________

13. Did rider or horse fall:

neither fell	rider fell	horse fell	both fell	not known
☐ 1	☐ 2	☐ 3	☐ 4	☐

14. Was the rider:

not injured	injured	killed	not known
☐ 1	☐ 2	☐ 3	☐

15. Did the rider consult a:

GP/Doctor	hospital	none	not known
☐ 1	☐ 2	☐ 3	☐

16. Was/were other road user(s):

not injured	injured	killed	not known
☐ 1	☐ 2	☐ 3	☐

no other road users involved ☐ 4 *(if no other road users involved answer question 18 go to question 21*

17. Did the other road user(s) consult a:

GP/Doctor	hospital	none	not known
☐ 1	☐ 2	☐ 3	☐

18. Was the horse:

not injured	injured	killed	not known
☐ 1	☐ 2	☐ 3	☐

19. Which part of horse did vehicle hit:

front	side	behind	not known	no collision
☐ 1	☐ 2	☐ 3	☐	☐ 4

other ☐ 5 specify ______________

20. Was the vehicle damaged:

no	not serious	serious	not known
☐ 1	☐ 2	☐ 3	☐

21. Age of rider:

under 12	12–16	19–30	31–64	65+	not known	no rider involved
☐ 1	☐ 2	☐ 3	☐ 4	☐ 5	☐	☐ 6

22. Sex of rider:

male	female	not known	no rider involved
☐ 1	☐ 2	☐	☐ 3

23. Type of area:

city	town	suburb	village	countryside	not known
☐ 1	☐ 2	☐ 3	☐ 4	☐ 5	☐

24. Type of road:

dual carriageway	main	minor	not known	not on road
☐ 1	☐ 2	☐ 3	☐	☐ 4

25. Which of the following statements best describes the accident:

Horse shied from shadow, bird etc and was hit by vehicle(s) .... ☐ 1
Horse frightened by one vehicle and hit by other(s) .... ☐ 2
Horse frightened and hit by same vehicle(s) .... ☐ 3
Horse frightened by vehicle(s) but not hit .... ☐ 4
Horse shied from shadow, bird etc and not hit by vehicle(s) .... ☐ 5
No vehicle involved .... ☐ 6
Details not known .... ☐
Horse escaped into traffic and hit by vehicle(s) .... ☐ 8
Other (please specify) .... ☐ 7

____

Give brief details of accident:

____
____
____
____

26. In what capacity are you filling in this form:

rider ☐ 1 motorist ☐ 2 witness ☐ 3 friend ☐ 4 police ☐ 5 relative ☐ 6

other ☐ 7 specify ____________

A representative of the British Horse Society may wish to obtain more details about this accident:

Your name: ______________________________

Your address: ______________________________
PLEASE PRINT ______________________________
____

Telephone No: daytime ______________ evening ______________

Please complete and send to:

THE SAFETY DEPARTMENT
THE BRITISH HORSE SOCIETY
STONELEIGH DEER PARK
KENILWORTH
WARWICKSHIRE CV8 2XZ

YOUR NAME AND ADDRESS WILL NOT BE ENTERED INTO THE COMPUTER

Thank you for completing this form.

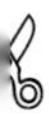

Authorised handbooks from The British Horse Society

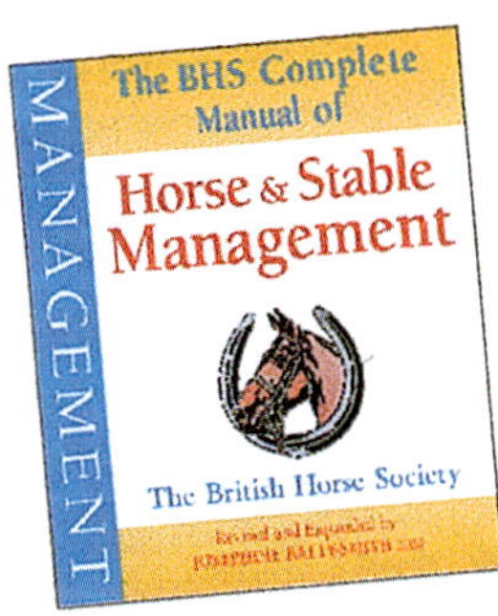

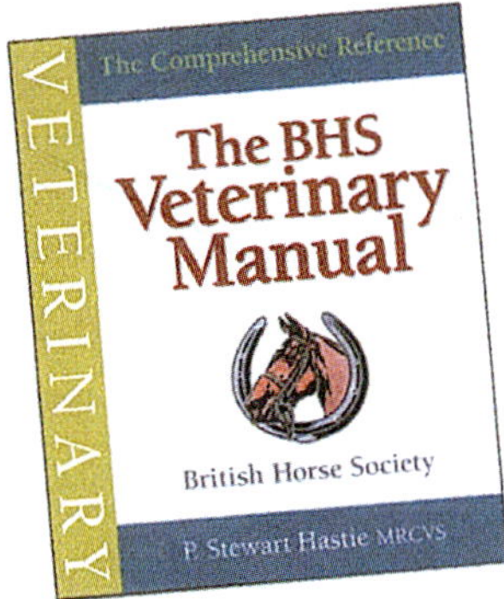

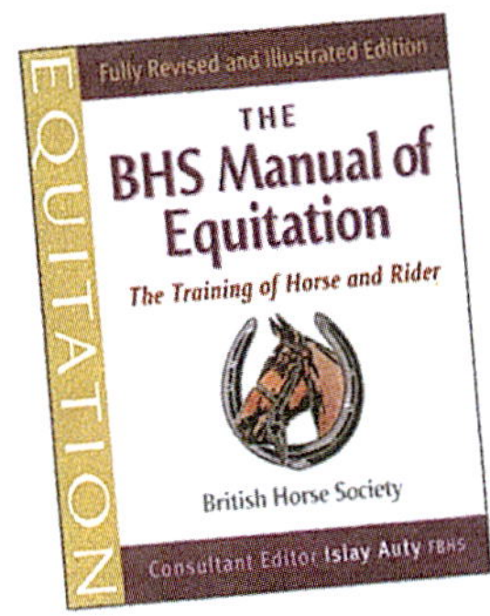

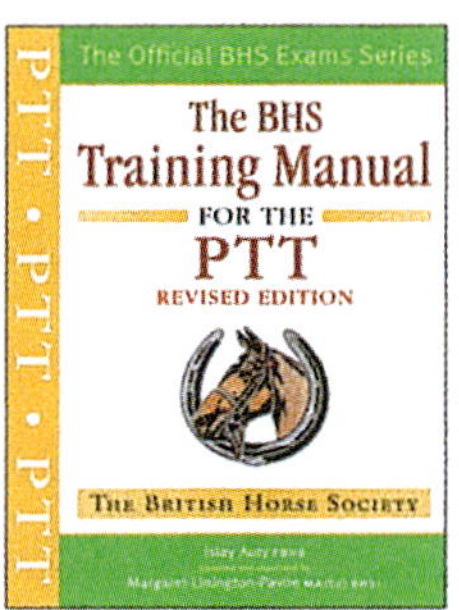

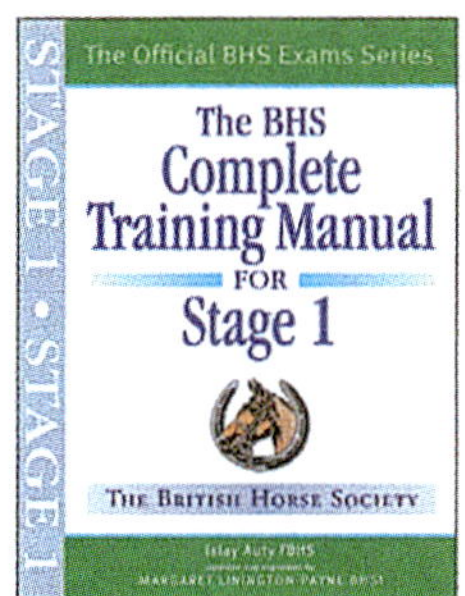

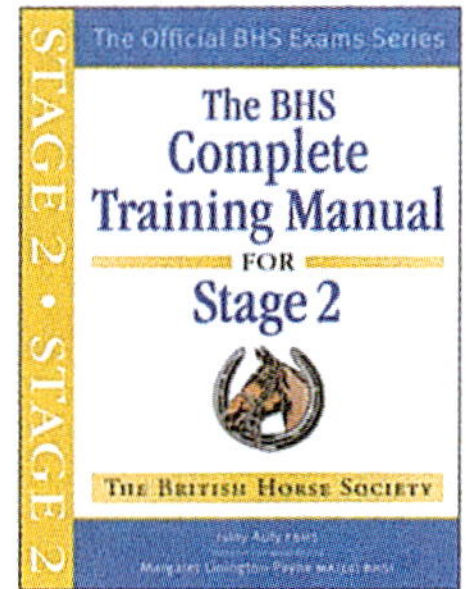

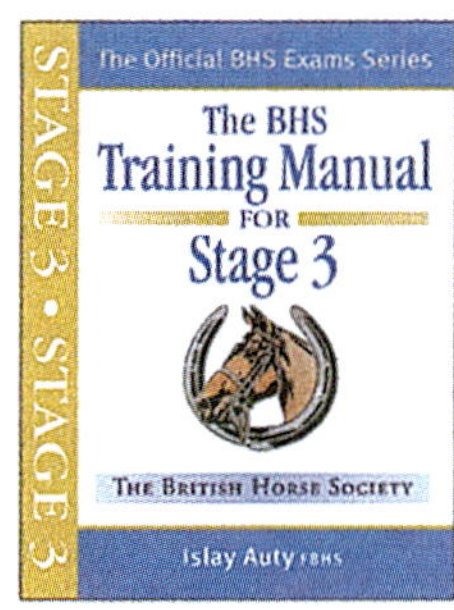

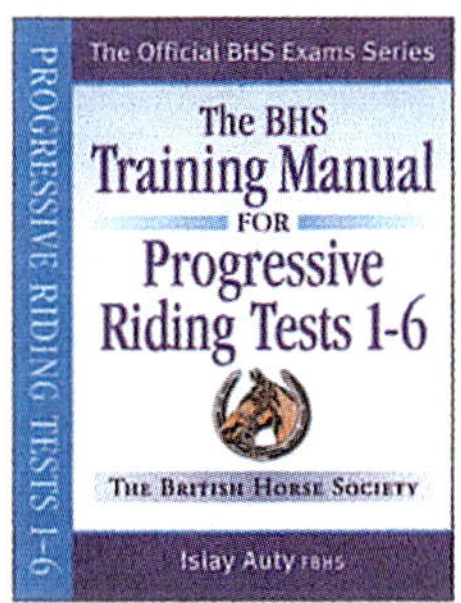

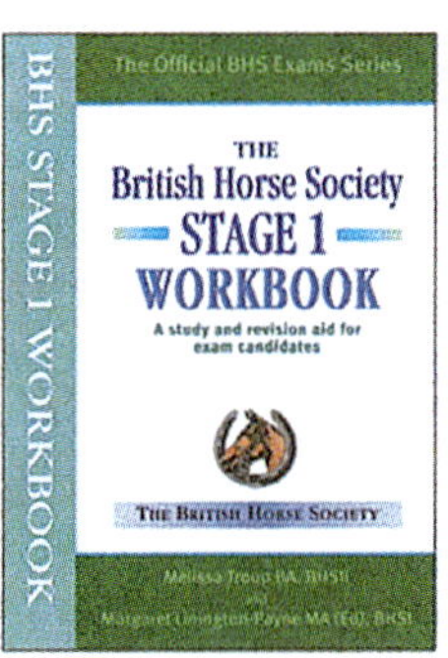

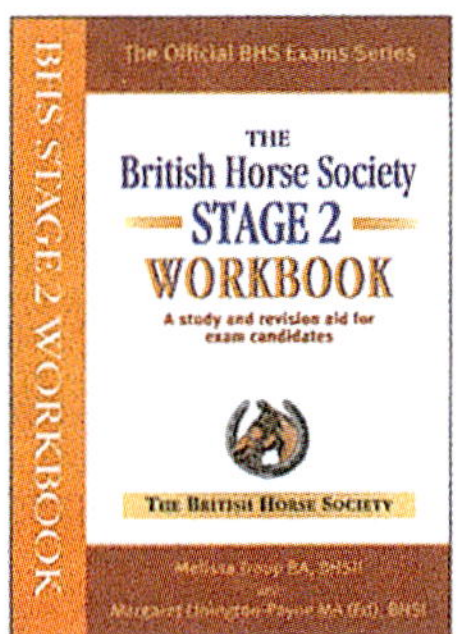

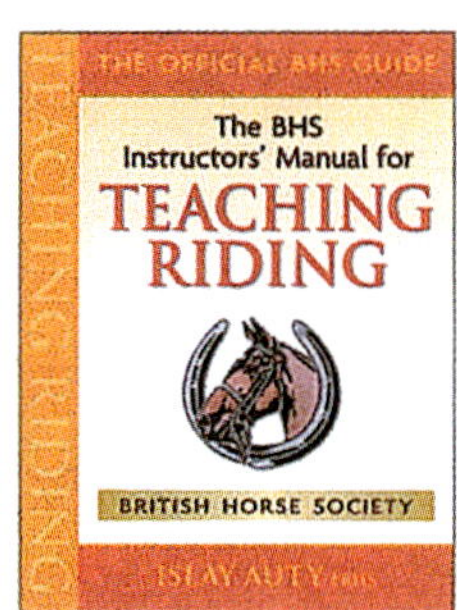

Obtainable from bookshops and saddlers and from

The British Horse Society Bookshop
Stoneleigh Deer Park
Stoneleigh
Warwickshire CV8 2XZ
Tel: 0844 848 1660 or visit the website - www.britishhorse.com